This Book Belongs To:

_____

THE
Little Book
of
YOGA

CHRONICLE BOOKS
SAN FRANCISCO

Library of Congress Cataloging-in-Publication Data:
Isaacs, Nora.
  The little book of yoga / text by Nora Isaacs.
    pages cm
  Includes index.
  ISBN 978-1-4521-2920-4 (alk. paper)
1. Hatha yoga. I. Title.
  RA781.7.I83 2014
  613.7'046—dc23

Manufactured in China

MIX
Paper from
responsible sources
FSC® C008047
www.fsc.org

Design by Tatiana Pavlova
Text by Nora Isaacs
Illustrations by Agnes Lee

The information, practices, and poses in this book are not offered as medical advice
or suggested as treatment for any condition that might require medical attention. To
avoid injury, practice yoga with a skilled instructor and consult a health professional to
determine your body's needs and limitations. The writer and publisher hereby disclaim
any liability from injuries resulting from following any recommendation in this book.

10 9 8 7 6

Chronicle Books LLC
680 Second Street
San Francisco, California 94107
www.chroniclebooks.com

CONTENTS

Introduction

The word *yoga* means "to unite." But what exactly are we bringing together when we bend, stretch, twist, and breathe?

The ancient yogis—a "yogi" being one who practices yoga—had some big ideas about union. They believed yoga could unite individuals with the universe, bring about the understanding that all beings are one, and enable us to experience total bliss. Most modern yogis don't have such lofty goals. We simply want to live more comfortably in our bodies. We want to be kinder, to feel better and more alive.

Practicing yoga is really very simple. You focus on your breath. You arrange your body like a cobra or a tree. You balance the best that you can. Yoga can strengthen your muscles, increase flexibility and circulation, boost your immunity, and calm your nervous system. But it can also strengthen your spirit. With a regular yoga practice, you become less reactive in stressful times. You blow off criticism more easily. You stand your ground more firmly. You start to notice the way the light shines through your window in the late afternoon. And you feel spontaneous moments of gratitude during an otherwise mundane moment, or a stirring of compassion for the people around you.

How does this work? How does physical exercise—something you might do to lose weight or build muscle—become something else entirely? It starts when you realize you can quiet your mind with your body. When you lie down calmly on your mat, you learn how to truly relax. When you fall down in a balancing pose, you learn that you can survive through—and even laugh at—your failures. When you ever so slowly stretch into a forward bend, you learn how to stay present. When you pay exquisite attention to each toe in a standing pose, you learn awareness. These benefits follow you off your mat and weave themselves into your daily life.

According to ancient yoga philosophy, every person is compassionate, loving, and peaceful. Yoga helps us uncover the basic goodness in ourselves and in others, which can so easily become buried beneath anger, resentment, self-criticism, and doubt. The more you practice yoga, the more clearly you can see the truth: All is as it should be. You are perfect just as you are.

This book invites you to learn more about yoga, offering general overviews and inspirational takeaways of various aspects of the tradition: the history, which spans ages and continents; the poses, including a selection of more than thirty-five common favorites; the philosophy, with explanations and present-day interpretations of each limb of the ancient yogi's guide to enlightenment, called the Eight-Limbed Path; related wellness exercises such as breathing, meditation, and mindfulness; and ideas for incorporating yoga into your daily life.

No matter what your skill level, and no matter what your goals—be they fitness-oriented, part of a larger spiritual quest, or tied to a simple curiosity about one of the world's great ancient traditions—there is always more to be learned about this mind-body practice. It's called a yoga "practice" because it's never quite finished. The wise yogi knows that the process itself is the destination. That life itself—perhaps even this very moment—is the ultimate reward. Discover these possibilities for yourself inside *The Little Book of Yoga.*

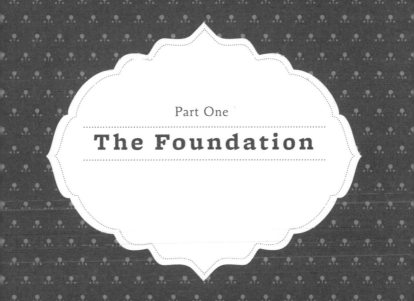

Part One

The Foundation

A Brief History of Yoga

The history of yoga is a complex web of branches and schools that twist and turn, leading to what is considered to be today's modern yoga. No one can pinpoint precisely when yoga was invented, but here's what we do know: Yoga hails from India. The language of yoga is called Sanskrit, an ancient priestly tongue. A pose is called an *asana*, based on the Sanskrit word for "seat." The yoga lifestyle has changed quite a bit since ancient times, when yogis lived in secluded caves or forests and practiced ways to master their bodies, such as stopping their heartbeat. But the essence of yoga remains the same, as does the ultimate goal: to find harmony with yourself and the world.

The Ancient Age

(3000 BCE–300 BCE)

Some scholars believe the yoga tradition began as early as 5,000 years ago, linking its origins to a soapstone seal, which was excavated in the early 1900s, that had human-like figures carved in shapes that looked like yoga poses. Others believe yoga is 2,500 years old, which is when it was first mentioned in an ancient text. Still others believe that yoga originated during the Vedic Age in India, when people focused on ritual, poetry, and transcending the mind through intense focus. During this time, holy men and women were said to have magical powers and practiced strenuous physical feats to overcome the body, which they considered an obstacle to enlightenment. These early yogis were committed to understanding their relationship with the divine, a core idea that is found in many schools of yoga today, thousands of years later.

Over time, the focus shifted from study and rituals toward self-understanding through direct experience. The body was no longer considered an obstacle; rather, it was seen as a means to finding freedom.

The Classical Age

(300 BCE–500 CE)

In yoga's Classical Age, which also took place in India, yoga came to be seen as a spiritual philosophy that could help people reach their full human potential. Finding freedom wasn't so much about uniting with some great spirit in the sky, but about awakening to one's own authentic self. It's known as the Classical Age because during this time, six classical philosophies were established, one of which is Patanjali's yoga. During this era, the emphasis of the practice was on meditation, rather than on yoga's physical poses.

HISTORIC TEXT OF THE CLASSICAL AGE: *The Yoga Sutra*
The Yoga Sutra is an authoritative text of the Classical Age. It was written at the dawn of the first millennium by a sage named Patanjali. It contains 196 aphorisms on the meaning of yoga, the experience of yoga, the expanding of one's yoga practice, and how yoga can free the soul. It also defined a set of guidelines called the Eight-Limbed Path (see page 134) that serves as a template for some modern-day yoga schools. And it identified five causes of suffering, called *kleshas*, which stand in the way of enlightenment. The five *kleshas* are ignorance (*avidya*), ego (*asmita*), attachment (*raga*), aversion to pain (*dvesa*), and fear of death (*abhinivesah*).

• 15TH–18TH CENTURIES •

The Foundational Texts on Yoga's Physical Poses

There are three key texts that describe yoga poses, breathing techniques, and meditation, which are the main practices of Hatha yoga, the most popular form of yoga practiced today. These foundational texts are the *Hatha Yoga Pradipika* (from the fifteenth century), the *Gheranda Samhita* (from the seventeenth century), and the *Shiva Samhita* (from the eighteenth century).

The Modern Age

(1893–PRESENT)

Modern yoga as we know it gained traction in the late 1800s after a few individual Indian yogis shared teachings of Eastern philosophy with Western audiences. Among those was Swami Vivekananda, a Hindu monk who gave an influential speech at the World Parliament of Religions in Chicago in 1893. Over the next century, more Indian teachers came to America, including B.K.S. Iyengar, Pattabhi Jois, Indra Devi, and T.K.V. Desikachar. These teachers, all students of a great Indian master called Krishnamacharya, went on to create the major styles practiced by today's yogis. Another Indian teacher, Paramahansa Yogananda, came to Boston in 1920 and founded the Self-Realization Fellowship. His book, *Autobiography of a Yogi*, is a wildly popular spiritual classic.

By the 1960s, yoga had taken hold in Western counter-culture. An Indian guru named Swami Satchidananda gave the opening speech at Woodstock in 1969, while the Beatles started traveling to India to study with a guru named Maharishi Mahesh Yogi. Ram Dass wrote a famous book called *Be Here Now* that heralded in the age of spiritual seekers. By the 1990s, yoga's popularity had fully transitioned from counterculture to the mainstream, where it thrives today.

HISTORIC TEXT OF THE MODERN AGE: *Light on Yoga*
Written by B.K.S. Iyengar and first published in 1966, *Light on Yoga* is considered to be the definitive manual on modern yoga. It includes descriptions and photographs of the yoga master himself in a wide range of poses. Iyengar went on to create an eponymous style of yoga, which focuses on precise alignment and the use of props.

The Branches of Yoga

What opens your heart? What makes you feel receptive to new ideas, creative, and compassionate? The many branches of yoga reflect the diversity of our temperaments, goals, and individual personalities. Whether it's rigorous exercise that opens one's heart, or music, or service to others, there's a branch of yoga for everyone, be it a traditional branch or a unique combination of many. Here are the modern forms of today's most relevant branches:

- BHAKTI YOGA (Devotion)
- HATHA YOGA (Physical Exercise)
- JNANA YOGA (Wisdom)
- KARMA YOGA (Service)
- MANTRA YOGA (Sound)
- RAJA YOGA (Meditation)

Bhakti Yoga

[THE YOGA OF DEVOTION]

Goal: To develop a personal relationship with the "divine," which could include a higher power, nature, or the self

How to get there: Prayer, chanting, or one's own preferred ways of expressing devotion

Common personality traits of a Bhakti yogi: Committed, sincere, strong in faith

Hatha Yoga

[THE YOGA OF PHYSICAL EXERCISE]

Goal: To gain freedom through physical discipline

How to get there: Do yoga poses to purify and prepare your body and mind

Common personality traits of a Hatha yogi: Active and energetic; enjoys a physical challenge

Jnana Yoga

[THE YOGA OF WISDOM]

Goal: To understand the truth though intense study and debate

How to get there: Read, study, analyze

Common personality traits of a Jnana yogi: Intellectual, philosophical, drawn to pursuits of the mind

Karma Yoga

[THE YOGA OF SERVICE]

Goal: To selflessly help others

How to get there: Volunteer work, public service, adopting a cause

Common personality traits of a Karma yogi: Generous, selfless, altruistic

Mantra Yoga

[THE YOGA OF SOUND]

Goal: To focus the mind using sound

How to get there: Chant a *mantra*, or repeat a chosen sound to reach a higher state of being

Common personality traits of a Mantra yogi: Focused, musical; appreciates solitude

Raja Yoga

[THE YOGA OF MEDITATION]

Goal: To clear the mind in order to experience moments of peace and clarity

How to get there: Cultivate a consistent meditation practice

Common personality traits of a Raja yogi: Curious, scientific, drawn to direct experience

Yoga Styles

When yoga hit the West in the late nineteenth century, a natural evolution occurred. Teachers trained by Indian masters began taking what they had learned and making it their own. Some instructors opened schools that followed closely in their particular lineage, while others used their knowledge as a starting point to develop their own creative styles. These days, there's a wide range of yoga styles suited to all personalities and skill levels, with variations in speed, levels of exertion, purposes, benefits, and environment (such as temperature of the room and noise level, for example).

Today's most popular styles include:

· ANUSARA YOGA
· ASHTANGA YOGA
· BIKRAM YOGA
· IYENGAR YOGA
· JIVAMUKTI YOGA
· KRIPALU YOGA
· KUNDALINI YOGA
· POWER YOGA
· RESTORATIVE YOGA
· VINIYOGA

Anusara Yoga

Anusara yoga presents the idea that, when practiced with proper alignment and intention, the poses can help one connect with inner joy, creativity, playfulness, and one's full potential. (As interpreted by Anusara yogis, the Sanskrit word *anusara* means "flowing with grace.") Rather than focusing on what needs to be fixed or corrected, Anusara teachers focus on the thriving goodness within and around us, and seek to help uncover each student's unique, innate beauty. Anusara's Universal Principles of Alignment, which incorporate yoga philosophy and physical alignment techniques, are applied to the teaching of each pose. Classes include an opening invocation, a heart-opening theme, a flowing sequence chosen from a selection of more than 250 poses, and a final relaxation period.

Ashtanga Yoga

Ashtanga yoga, founded by K. Pattabhi Jois (1915–2009), features flowing movements called *vinyasas* that connect breath with movement. When done correctly, the blood circulates freely, creating internal heat and sweating, which is believed to purify the body and calm the mind. Sometimes referred to as Ashtanga Vinyasa Yoga, this style follows a universal sequence that students gradually learn from their teacher as they progress in skill and ability. Classes open with Sun Salutations (see pages 38–39), followed by standing poses, seated poses, backbends, inversions, and finally a relaxation pose. The breath is central to this practice. Ashtanga incorporates audible throat breathing called *Ujjayi* (oo-JAH-ee) breath, which sounds like the ocean as the practitioner breathes in and out, evenly and in rhythm with the movements of the body. Ashtanga also incorporates *bandhas* (see page 178), or internal body locks that are thought to gather energy in the body, and *drishti*, a focused gaze. Flow yoga and vinyasa yoga are variations of Ashtanga yoga.

Bikram Yoga

Bikram yoga, founded by Bikram Choudhury (b. 1946), is a standardized series of twenty-six poses practiced in a room heated to 105°F/40°C. The heat is believed to release toxins, improve circulation, and loosen up muscles. Because of the heat, it's recommended that you dress lightly, and bring a towel and a bottle of water. The practice starts and ends with breathing exercises and includes standing poses, backbends, seated poses, and twists. Each pose is done twice, and proceeds in a fixed order. It's often called Hot Yoga when there is some deviation from Bikram's prescribed sequence.

Iyengar Yoga

Iyengar yoga was founded by B.K.S. Iyengar (b. 1918), who considered the body to be a vehicle toward a spiritual path. This style emphasizes precise alignment, anatomy, and sequencing of the poses in a very specific order. Classes are conducted like an in-depth workshop, focusing on only a few poses, hands-on adjustments, and holding demonstrations in the center of the room. Iyengar yoga encourages the use of props like blocks, chairs, blankets, and bolsters to promote relaxation, proper alignment, and opening the body in a safe way. Those who are sensitive to injury, or are healing from a specific injury, find Iyengar useful because of the careful instructions, attention to body mechanics, and thoughtful modifications of the poses to suit individual needs and comfort preferences.

Jivamukti Yoga

Jivamukti yoga, founded in New York City by Sharon Gannon and David Life in 1986, is a rigorous form of flowing yoga. Energetic Jivamukti classes include Sun Salutations, poses, chanting, music, relaxation, and meditation. Some classes open with a theme that is woven throughout the class, and there is an emphasis on alignment and hands-on adjustment. Loosely translated from Sanskrit, *jivan mukti* means "liberation while living." The founders' philosophy centers around five tenets: kindness, devotion, meditation, music, and studying yoga scripture. They encourage practitioners to bring yoga philosophy off the mat and into their daily lives, and to live in a kind and compassionate way.

Kripalu Yoga

Kripalu yoga was founded by Amrit Desai (b. 1932), a native of India who was inspired by Swami Kripalvananda (1913–1981), after whom the practice is named. With a focus on bringing awareness to poses, breathwork, and meditation, Kripalu yoga encourages healing, psychological growth, spirituality, and creativity. By focusing on staying in the present moment while on the mat, this style encourages deepening your spiritual attunement, self-awareness, and empathy. It combines a slow-moving yet challenging class with a meditative awareness. Kripalu employs an approach referred to as BRFWA: breathe, relax, feel, watch, and allow. These five steps can be applied to everyday life as part of a practice of self-acceptance.

Kundalini Yoga

Kundalini yoga practices—including breathing, poses, hand positions, chanting, and meditation—are designed to awaken the latent energy that sits at the base of the spine, so that one can experience a higher consciousness. The practices focus on balancing the glandular and nervous systems for physical, mental, and spiritual health. A chant often heard in a Kundalini yoga class is *Sat Nam*, which means "truth is my identity." Kundalini yoga, as inspired by Yogi Bhajan (1929–2004), encourages teachers and practitioners to wear white clothing to nourish light and divinity.

Power Yoga

Power yoga is an overarching term for an athletic style of yoga that is popular in a gym setting as well as in studios. Its roots are in Ashtanga yoga. Poses are linked together by a *chaturanga* pose (see page 51), and movements flow swiftly for an often sweaty cardio workout, likely accompanied by upbeat music. Variations of Power yoga are Power Vinyasa Flow, Dynamic Yoga, and Power Vinyasa.

Restorative Yoga

Restorative yoga is designed to counter stress by triggering the parasympathetic nervous system, which calms the body and lowers heart rate and blood pressure. Restorative yoga poses often incorporate props such as bolsters, blocks, and blankets that completely support the body, allowing it to relax and drop deeply into a stress-free state. Each pose requires time for the practitioner to arrange the body and adjust props until they arrive in a position of complete comfort. Once there, they lie still for up to 20 minutes. Restorative yoga was popularized by Judith Hanson Lasater—a physical therapist, yoga teacher, and scholar—in the 1990s.

Viniyoga

Viniyoga is useful for all kinds of yogis, and is often recommended for people with injuries or illness because it's highly adaptable to one's needs. The practice includes poses, breathwork, meditation, chanting, and other methods designed to transform the body and mind. In a Viniyoga class, one might move in and out of the same pose repeatedly, making slight modifications while also focusing on the breath. Viniyoga was shaped by Gary Kraftsow (b. 1955), who based the practice on the teachings of Krishnamacharya (1888–1989) and T.K.V. Desikachar (b. 1938).

················· **What Is Hatha Yoga?** ·················

Hatha yoga refers specifically to the physical aspect of yoga. The word *hatha* in Sanskrit means "force," which can describe the strengthening movements of the body during a yoga class. Historically, physical movement was just one small part of the larger yoga tradition, but today the physical exercises known as Hatha yoga are what many recognize as modern yoga. Classes described as "hatha" often blend a few different styles rather than emphasizing just one.

················· **What Is Vinyasa Yoga?** ·················

Some modern yoga classes are referred to as "vinyasa yoga," which means that poses are linked together with flowing movements, and often linked to the breath. Vinyasa also refers to carefully thought-out sequencing, with one pose preparing the body for the next. Think of vinyasa as a graceful dance, with the same moves being repeated continuously.

Part Two

Yoga Poses

Yoga poses are the building blocks of a physical yoga practice, and a gateway into a deeper understanding of the mind and body. Traditionally, yoga poses—of which there was only a small selection in ancient times—were done in preparation for seated meditation, helping to strengthen the back and core and open up the hips to facilitate long periods of sitting (see *asana*, the third limb of the Eight-Limbed Path, page 140). Today, having been adapted by modern society into a flourishing type of exercise, they feature prominently in a range of fitness and wellness programs and are enjoyed for their myriad health benefits, mental and physical.

True to their origins, most yoga poses have a Sanskrit name that ends with *asana*—such as *Savasana* (page 129) or *Bhujangasana* (page 109)—which means "seat." Poses are often named for animals and objects whose shapes and characteristics inspire the pose, such as a cobra, boat, and warrior. They are often categorized by the basic positioning of the body: standing, balancing, seated, resting, plus backbends and inversions.

With hundreds of poses to choose from, a yoga practice is infinitely customizable for every skill level, personality, and wellness goal. Yoga poses can be the center of a fitness program or can be an occasional add-on. Individually or grouped together, they can target specific muscles and areas of the body. Strung together into dynamic sequences, they can provide a full-body workout. A group class can be an energizing, communal experience, while practice on one's own can instill discipline and serenity. Fast and rigorous, or slow and soothing, it's the participant's choice and the options are endless.

The benefits are as diverse as the poses themselves. Practitioners say that yoga can attune the body and mind, boost circulation, and support the body's digestive, nervous, and hormonal systems. Physical benefits can include increased strength and flexibility. Mental benefits can range from improved sleep to balanced moods, and overall enhanced well-being. Over time, a yoga practice can naturally lead to healthier eating habits and lifestyle changes that might have once seemed unrealistic. It can even bring about a gentle spiritual awakening as self-acceptance and peaceful intentions are emphasized with each stretch, flex, and twist of the body.

The following pages present a sampling of some of the most commonly taught yoga poses, ideal for mixing, matching, and modifying to suit anyone's wellness goals.

Sun Salutation

Yoga's classic Sun Salutation (*Surya Namaskar*, in Sanskrit) is a flowing sequence that awakens the body and mind. Do it two times briskly on each side, linking each movement with your breath, for an energizing way to greet the day.

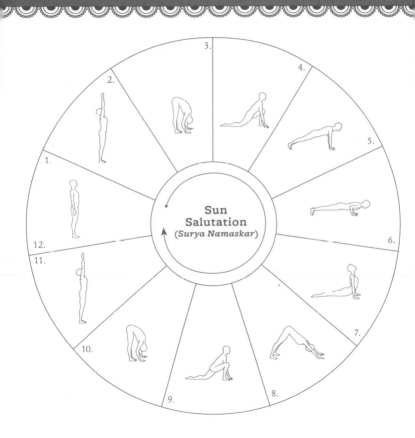

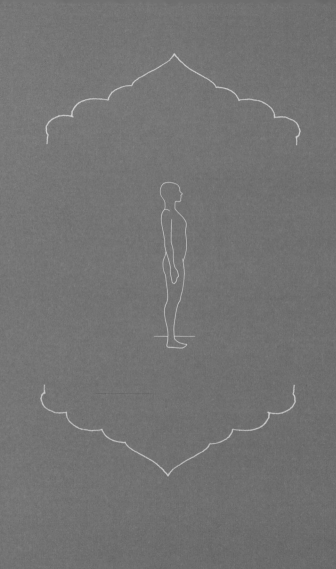

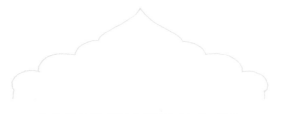

MOUNTAIN POSE

TADASANA
(ta-DA-sah-nah)

Origin: *Tada* means "mountain."

How to do it: Stand with your feet together, with the big toes and heels touching. Keep your feet relaxed. Bring your arms alongside your body, palms facing your thighs. Keep your head and spine in a straight line, one atop the other.

Benefits: Increases body awareness.

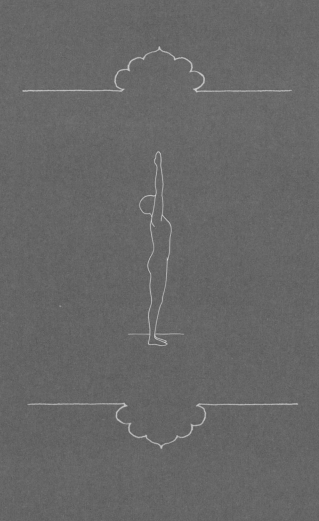

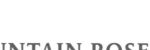

MOUNTAIN POSE
WITH ARMS UP

How to do it: Stand with your feet together, with the big toes and heels touching. Keep your feet relaxed. Inhale as your bring your arms overhead, palms touching. Look up at your hands and slightly bend back from your waist.

Benefits: Stretches the front and sides of the body.

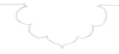

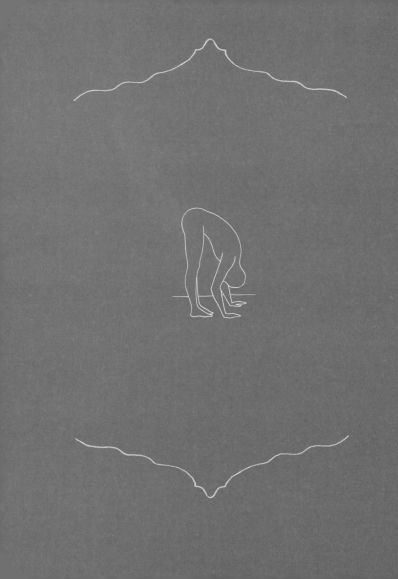

STANDING
FORWARD BEND

How to do it: Stand with your feet together, with the big toes and heels touching. Keep your feet relaxed. Exhale as you bring your arms out to the sides and bend from your hips, diving forward. Bring your palms to the floor in front of you. If they don't reach, bend your knees or let your arms hang. Relax your head toward the floor.

Benefits: Stretches the hamstrings, spine, and neck.

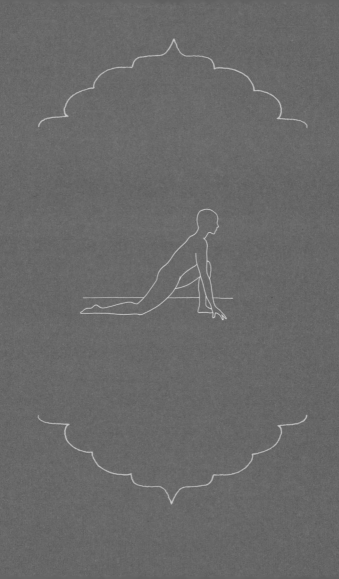

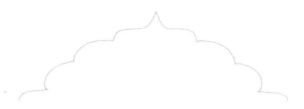

LUNGE

How to do it: Stand with your feet together, with the big toes and heels touching. Keep your feet relaxed. Bring one foot back into a lunge, with the knee of that leg resting on the floor behind you, and the other knee at a right angle with the mat.

Benefits: Strengthens the legs.

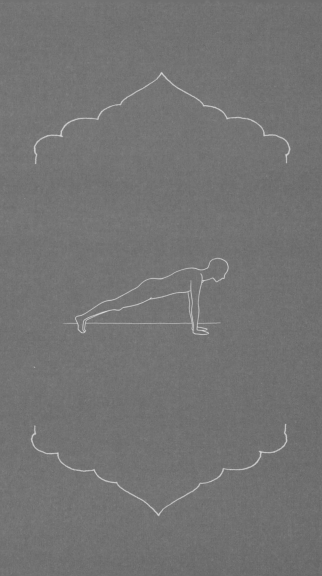

PLANK POSE

How to do it: Starting with your knees on your mat,
lean forward and place your hands flat on the mat
in front of you. Straighten your legs, tuck your toes
under, and shift your weight onto your toes and hands,
so your knees rise off the mat. Bring your body into
a straight diagonal line from the top of your head to
your heels. Avoid locking your arms; keep them very
slightly bent. Bring back your shoulders so your heart
lifts slightly, and press firmly into the floor with your
palms, while maintaining energy in your legs.

Benefits: Strengthens the arms, wrists,
and abdominals.

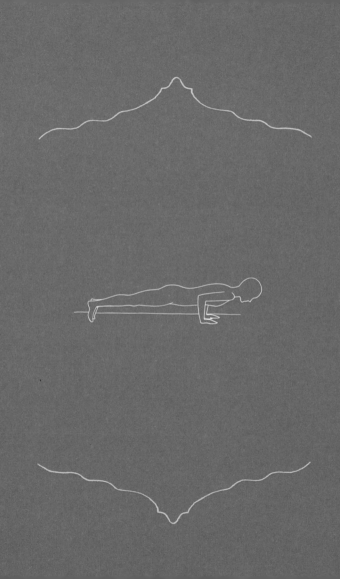

FOUR-LIMBED
STAFF POSE

CHATURANGA DANDASANA
(chat-ur-ANGA don-DAH-sah-nah)

Origin: *Chatur* means "four," *anga* means "limb,"
danda means "staff."

How to do it: From Plank Pose (see page 49), hug
your elbows toward your body. Keeping your body in a
straight line, lower yourself to just above your mat, so
your body is parallel with the floor. Press your hands
into the mat as you look slightly forward without
straining your neck.

Benefits: Strengthens the abdomen, arms, and wrists.

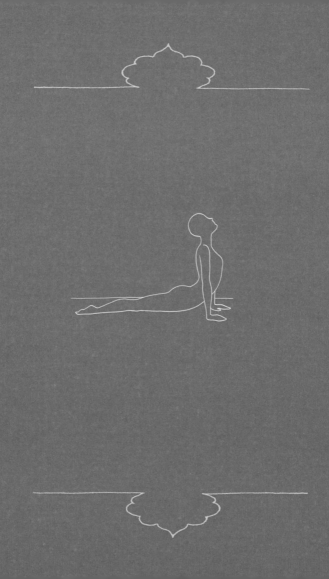

UPWARD-FACING DOG

URDHVA MUKHA SVANASANA
(OOrd-va MOO-ka svan-AH-sah-nah)

Origin: *Urdhva* means "upward," *mukha* means "face,"
svana means "dog."

How to do it: Lower your body onto the floor to rest
on your stomach, and place your hands beneath your
shoulders. Press your palms down into the mat, and
slowly lift your upper body off the floor by pressing into
your palms, opening your chest. If this is comfortable,
go deeper by straightening your arms so that your lower
body lifts, with only the tops of your feet touching the
floor. Keep your legs active and your buttocks relaxed.
Roll your shoulders back and down and open your chest
as you gaze forward or gently upward.

Benefits: Opens the front body and chest.
Strengthens the back.

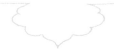

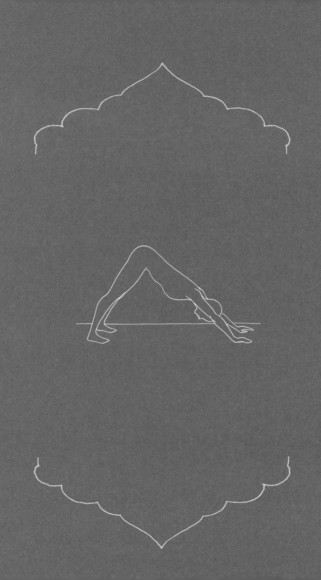

DOWNWARD-FACING DOG

ADHO MUKHA SVANASANA
(ODD-ho MOO-ka svan-AII-sah-nah)

Origin: *Adhomukha* means "face downward,"
svana means "dog."

How to do it: Start in Plank Pose (page 49). As you
inhale, lift your hips toward the sky so your body
forms two sides of a triangle, with your hips at the
highest point. Press your palms firmly into the floor,
and move your torso toward your thighs, lengthening
your spine and your breath.

Benefits: Stretches the hamstrings, ankles, shoulders,
and calves. Reduces stiffness in the shoulders.

Standing Poses

Standing poses set a strong foundation for your yoga practice and your life. By using the body's large muscles, you'll build overall strength, flexibility, and stamina. These poses require balance and grace, and help to build the confidence of a warrior.

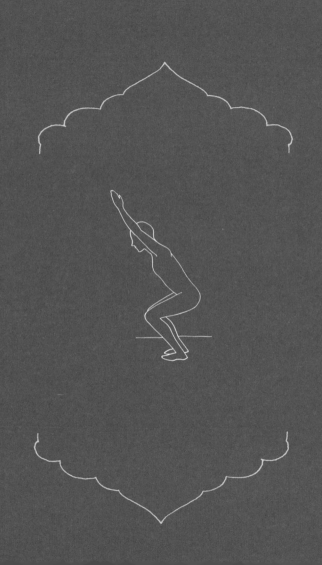

CHAIR POSE
(or FIERCE POSE)

UTKATASANA
(OOT-kah-TAH-sah-nah)

Origin: *Utkata* means "fierce."

How to do it: Stand with your feet together and your arms by your sides. Take a big breath in, then exhale and bend your knees deeply, like you're sitting in a chair. Reach your arms straight up in a gentle diagonal.

Benefits: Strengthens and tones the legs, gluteal muscles, and arms. Stretches the side body.

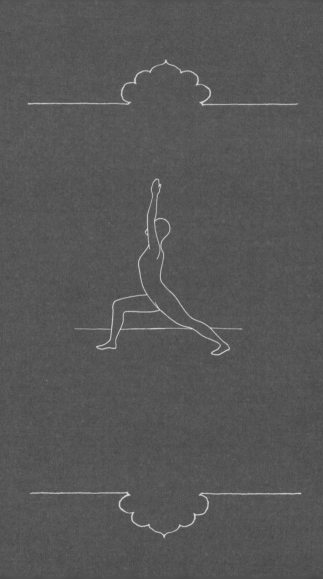

WARRIOR POSE I

VIRABHADRASANA I
(vee-rah-hah-DRAH-sah nah)

Origin: *Virabhadra* means "warrior."

How to do it: From Mountain Pose (page 41), step your feet wide apart. Turn your right foot out and your left foot slightly in. Square your hips toward your right foot. Inhale deeply and, as you exhale, bend your right knee, moving your right leg into a perpendicular angle, with your right thigh parallel with the floor (or as close as you can come while remaining comfortable). Reach your arms up alongside your ears and gaze softly forward. To deepen the pose, join your palms and gaze up at your thumbs. (Switch sides to work the opposite part of the body.)

Benefits: Strengthens the legs and ankles. Stretches the front of the hips, abdomen, hip flexors, and psoas. Strengthens the upper back.

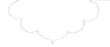

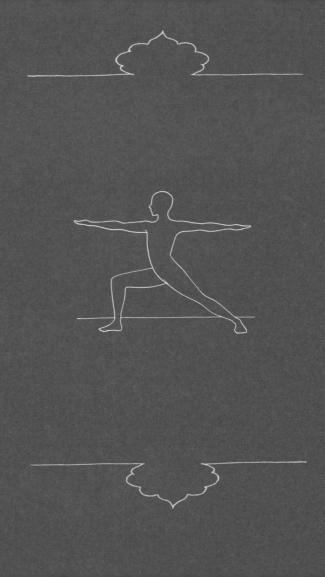

WARRIOR POSE II

VIRABHADRASANA II
(vee-rah-bah-DRAH-sah-nah)

Origin: *Virabhadra* means "warrior."

How to do it: From Mountain Pose (page 41), step
your feet wide apart and spread your arms out wide so
they are parallel with the floor. Turn your right foot
out to the right, and your left foot slightly in so the
toes point toward the right foot. Inhale deeply and, as
you exhale, bend your right knee, moving your right
leg into a perpendicular angle, with your right thigh
becoming parallel with the floor (or as close as you
can get while remaining comfortable). Turn your head
to gaze over your right hand. (Switch sides to work the
opposite part of the body.)

Benefits: Strengthens the legs, ankles, upper back,
and arms. Stretches the inner thighs.

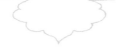

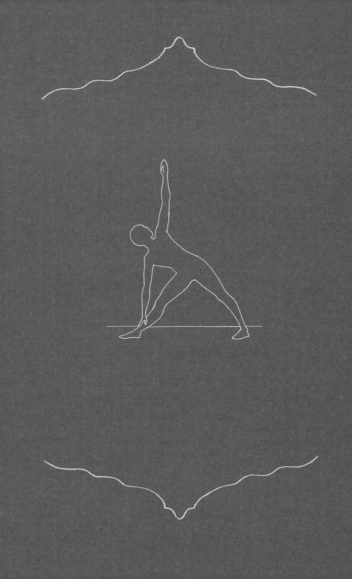

EXTENDED TRIANGLE POSE

UTTHITA TRIKONASANA
(oo-TEE-tah trik-cone-AH-sah-nah)

Origin: *Trikona* means "three angles" or "triangle."

How to do it: From Mountain Pose (page 41), step
your feet wide apart. Turn your right foot out and your
left foot slightly in. Inhale deeply and reach your arms
out wide so they are parallel with the floor, creating a
T-shape with your body. As you exhale, reach out to
the right, tilt downward at your waist, and place your
right hand lightly on your right shin. Lift your left
arm up to the sky, imagining a straight line all the
way from the right fingertips to the left fingertips.
Gaze up at your left thumb. (Switch sides to work the
opposite part of the body.)

Benefits: Strengthens and tones the legs. Stretches the
legs, hips, shoulders, and spine.

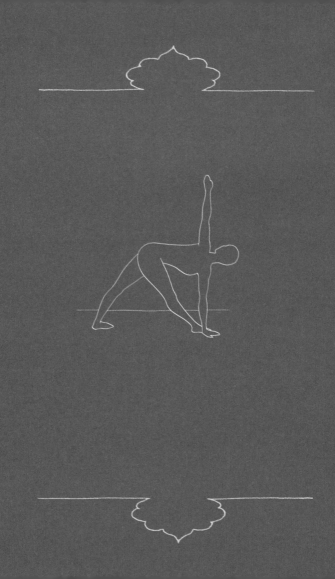

REVOLVED TRIANGLE POSE

PARIVRTTA TRIKONASANA
(pah-ree-VRIT-ah trik-cone AH-sah-nah)

Origin: *Parivrtta* means "to turn or revolve."

How to do it: From Mountain Pose (page 41), step your feet apart. Turn your right foot out and your left foot slightly in. Square your hips and align your heels with each other. Inhale as you place your right hand on your right hip, while your left hand reaches toward the sky. Exhale and bend over your front leg, placing your left hand at the outside of your right foot. Turn your chest up toward the sky and lift your right hand, imagining a straight line from the left fingertips all the way to the right fingertips. (Switch sides to work the opposite part of the body.)

Benefits: Stretches the side body, chest, and muscles around the spine. Strengthens and stretches the legs, ankles, and hips.

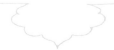

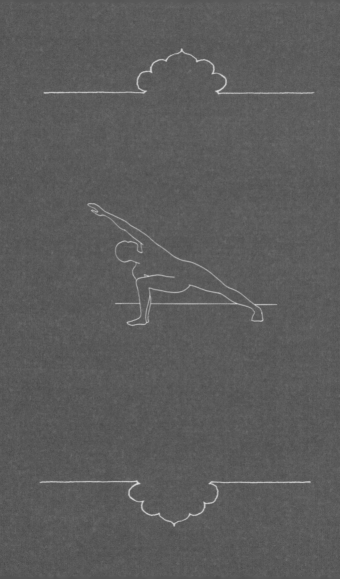

EXTENDED SIDE ANGLE POSE

UTTHITA PARSVAKONASANA
(oo-TEE-tah pars-vah-cone-AH-sah-nah)

Origin: *Utthita* means "to extend."

How to do it: From Mountain Pose (page 41), step your feet wide apart, with your feet parallel. Turn your right foot out, bend your right knee to 90 degrees, and turn your left foot slightly in toward your body. Tilting downward at your waist to place your right hand at the outside of your right foot, sweep your left arm up and alongside your left ear, creating a diagonal line from your left ankle all the way to your left fingertips. Keeping your gaze soft, look up under your left arm. (Switch sides to work the opposite part of the body.)

Benefits: Stretches the side body, chest, and muscles around the spine. Strengthens and stretches the legs, ankles, and hips.

Balancing Poses

These balancing poses sharpen concentration and teach lessons of perseverance, while increasing flexibility, and strengthening and toning the abdomen and legs.

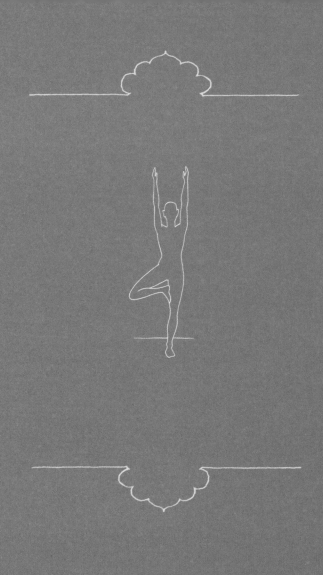

TREE POSE

VRKSASANA
(vrik-SHAHS-ah-nah)

Origin: *Vrksa* means "tree."

How to do it: From Mountain Pose (page 41), bring your weight onto your left foot. Breathing steadily, place the sole of your right foot either below your knee or as high up on your inner left thigh as you can, and keep it there. (For a less challenging alternative, stand next to a wall and place your hand on it for support.) When you have achieved a strong foundation standing on one foot, reach your arms toward the sky, "growing" like a tree. To take it farther, lift your gaze toward your hands. (Switch sides to work the opposite part of the body.)

Benefits: Improves balance. Strengthens the ankles and legs. Stretches the outer hips and inner thigh.

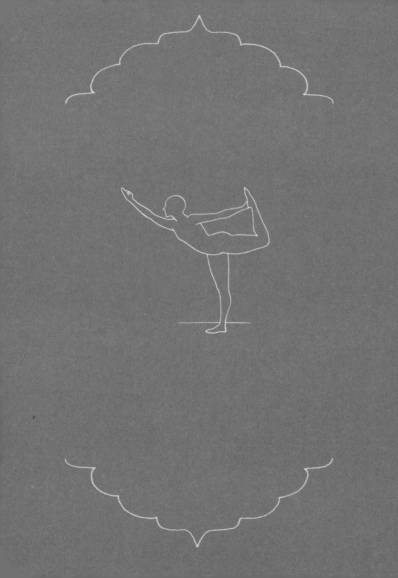

DANCER'S POSE

NATARAJASANA
(nah-tah-rah-JAHS-ah-nah)

Origin: The Hindu deity Nataraja is the dancing form of Lord Shiva.

How to do it: From Mountain Pose (page 41), bring your weight onto your right foot. Bend your left knee and bring your left heel toward your buttocks. Reach back with your left hand (using a wall for support, if needed) and gently grasp the inner arch of the foot. Breathe steadily as you reach forward with your right arm, tilting your body forward while simultaneously lifting your left leg back and up as it presses into your hand. (Switch sides to work the opposite part of the body.)

Benefits: Strengthens the legs, back, and abdominal muscles. Improves balance. Stretches the front of the hip and thigh, and the chest and shoulders.

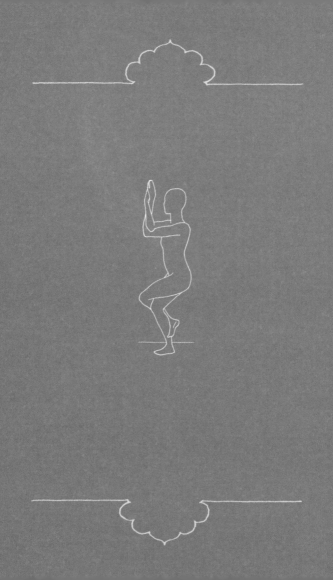

EAGLE POSE

GARUDASANA
(gah-roo-DAH-sah-nah)

Origin: *Garuda* means "eagle."

How to do it: From Mountain Pose (page 41), bend both knees and cross your left thigh over your right thigh. Bend the knees more deeply and deepen the twist of your legs by wrapping the top of your left foot around the back of your right calf. Holding the legs in this pose, inhale and reach both arms out in front of you. Then cross them in front of your body, right arm above left. Then bend your elbows and wrap your forearms into a twist until your left fingertips press against your right palm. Breathe steadily, holding the full-body pose as long as comfortable. (Switch sides to work the opposite part of the body.)

Benefits: Stretches and strengthens the ankles and legs. Stretches the shoulders, upper back, and hips. Improves balance.

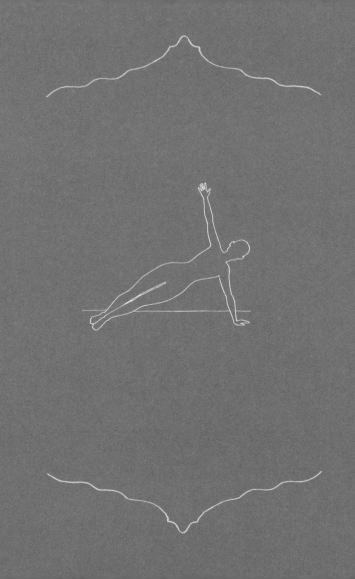

SIDE PLANK POSE

VASISTHASANA
(vah-see-STAHS-ah-nah)

Origin: This pose is dedicated to the sage Vasistha.

How to do it: Start with your weight on your hands and knees. Tuck your toes under and straighten your legs, coming into a push-up position. Roll your entire body to the left, in a counterclockwise position, until the outer edge of your left foot rests against the mat. Stack your right foot on top of your left foot so your legs are stacked as well. Engage your legs, tuck your tailbone under slightly, and reach your right arm up to the sky, so your whole body is supported only by your left hand and your left foot. To take it farther, gaze up at your right hand. (Switch sides to work the opposite part of the body.)

Benefits: Strengthens the side body, arms, legs, and abdominal muscles. Improves concentration and balance.

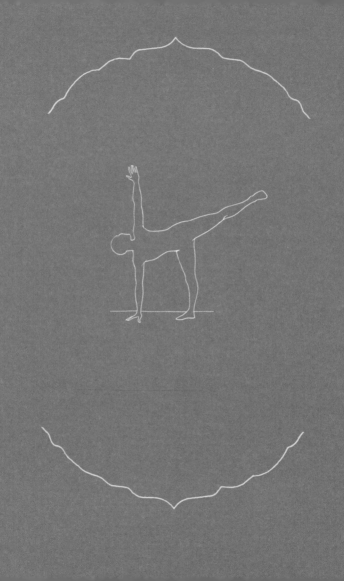

HALF MOON POSE

ARDHA CHANDRASANA
(ARE-duh chan-DRAH-sah-nah)

Origin: *Ardha* means "half," *chandra* means "moon."

How to do it: From Extended Triangle Pose (page 65), with your right leg forward, place your left hand on your left hip. Bend your right knee and slide your right fingertips forward, touching the floor. Once you achieve a strong foundation, straighten your right knee and lift your left leg off the ground, flexing your foot by pressing through your left heel. To take it farther, reach your left arm skyward and gaze up. (Switch sides to work the opposite part of the body.)

Benefits: Strengthens the legs, abdominals, and muscles around the spine. Builds balance.

Seated Poses, Twists, and Abdominal Strengtheners

Seated poses bring flexibility to the hips, legs, ankles, and groin, while twists keep the spine long and strong, and also apply circulation-boosting pressure to the abdominal organs. Abdominal strengtheners are key to building a strong core that powers a yoga practice.

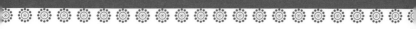

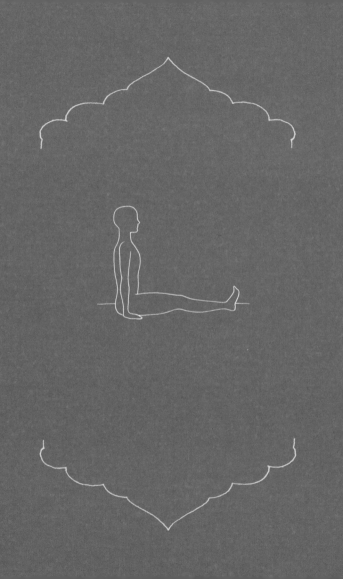

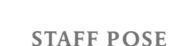

STAFF POSE

DANDASANA
(dahn-DAH-sah-nah)

Origin: *Danda* means "staff."

How to do it: Sit with your legs extended on your mat straight out in front of you. (If your back starts to round, sit on a cushion or folded blanket.) Place your palms on the floor alongside your outer hips. Press down through your palms, lengthening your spine as you sit taller (but without your legs or buttocks lifting off the floor). Breathe softly and fluidly.

Benefits: Encourages correct alignment of the spine and strengthens the supporting back muscles.

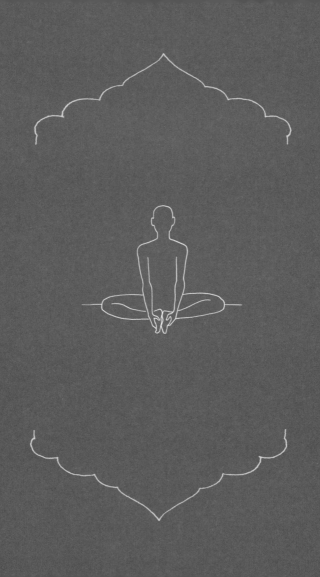

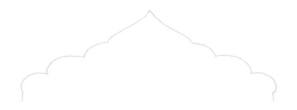

BOUND ANGLE POSE

BADDHA KONASANA
(BAH-dah cone-AH-sah-nah)

Origin: *Baddha* means "bound," *kona* means "angle."

How to do it: From Staff Pose (page 85), bend your knees and place the soles of your feet together. Allow your knees to drop open to the sides. Wrap your hands around the outer edges of your feet and press your thumbs into your foot arches. Root down through your seat and lift your chest. Feel your head floating above your long spine. Breathe softly and fluidly.

Benefits: Stretches the inner thighs and outer hips.

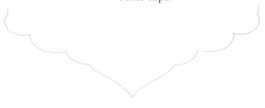

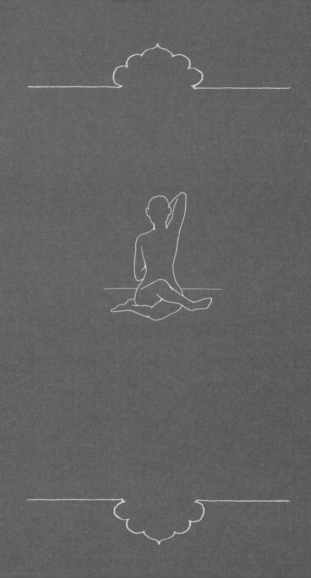

COW-FACE POSE

GOMUKHASANA
(GO-moo-KAH-sah-nah)

Origin: *Go* means "cow," *mukha* means "face."

How to do it: Start with your weight on your hands and knees. Slide your left knee behind your right knee so your feet are at either side of your body, and then sit back into the space between your feet so that your knees are stacked, one on top of the other. Reach your left arm up alongside your ear; bend that arm and rest the fingertips on your upper back. Stretch your right arm out to the right with the thumb pointing toward the ground. Bend the right elbow and place the back of your hand on your lower back. From here, you'll either move your hands toward each other until they touch, or keep your hands where they are. When comfortable, exhale as you gently bend forward over your legs. (Switch sides to work the opposite part of the body.)

Benefits: Stretches the hips and ankles. Stretches the shoulders, triceps, and chest.

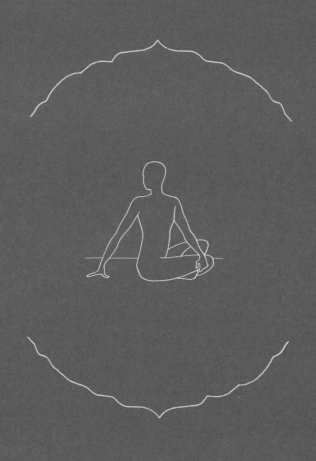

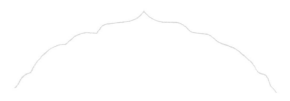

SEATED TWIST

How to do it: Sit in a cross-legged position, with one shin crossed over the other. Inhale and place your left hand on your right knee. Rest your right palm on the floor behind you. Exhale and gently twist, turning your gaze over your right shoulder. (Switch sides to work the opposite part of the body.)

Benefits: Gently wakes up and stretches the muscles around the spine. Stretches the outer hips.

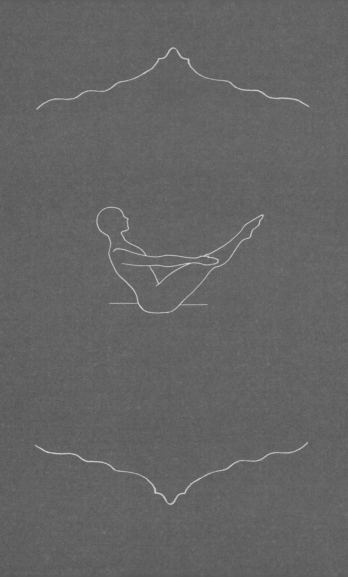

FULL BOAT POSE

PARIPURNA NAVASANA
(pah-ree-POOR-nah nah-VAH-sah-nah)

Origin: *Paripurna* means "full," *nava* means "boat."

How to do it: From Staff Pose (page 85), lean back, bend your knees, and draw them toward your chest, lifting your feet off the floor. Straighten your legs as far as you comfortably can, feeling your abdominal muscles engage. To go farther, reach your arms straight out in front of you, on either side of your outer thighs. Remain here, balancing on your buttocks, gazing at your toes, and breathing consciously and continuously.

Benefits: Strengthens the abdominal muscles, inner thighs, quadriceps, and hamstrings.

Forward Bends and Hip Openers

Forward bends are known for their calming qualities, inviting introspection and promoting stress reduction while at the same time strengthening the muscles along your spine. Hip openers alleviate back pain and reduce stress on the knees.

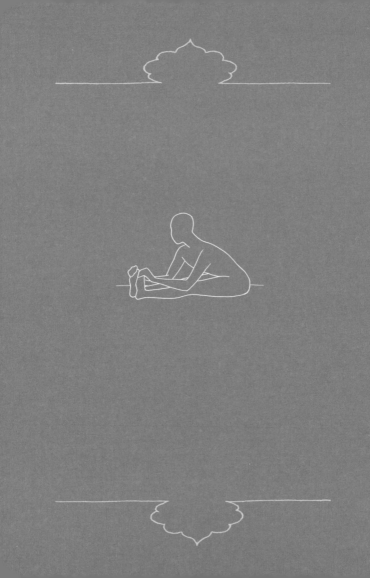

SEATED
FORWARD BEND

PASCHIMOTTANASANA
(PAH-she-mow-tahn-AH-sah-nah)

Origin: *Paschima* means "west," *uttana* means
"intense stretch." The pose is loosely translated as
"intense stretch of the west."

How to do it: From Staff Pose (page 85), inhale deeply
and lengthen your spine. Press your legs into the earth.
Flex your feet and reach your arms out in front of you.
Exhale and bend forward over your legs, going only as
far as you can without letting your spine bend out of its
taut length. (If your back rounds right away, sit up on
a folded blanket and re-attempt the pose.) If you can
reach them, grasp your feet with your hands. If not,
leave your arms reaching forward as far as they will go.

Benefits: Stretches the hamstrings and all of the
muscles up and down the back. Encourages proper
spinal alignment and posture.

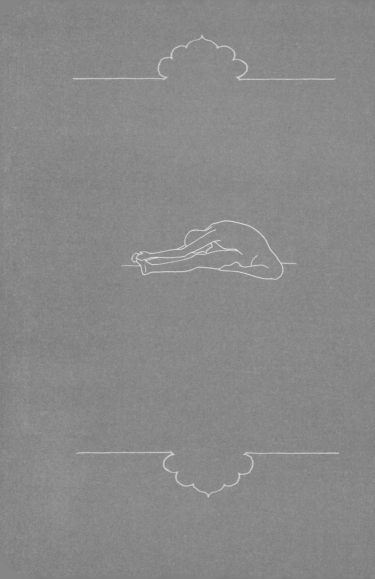

HEAD-TO-KNEE POSE

JANU SIRSASANA
(JAH-new shear-SHAH-sah-nah)

Origin: *Janu* means "knee," *sirsa* means "head."

How to do it: From Staff Pose (page 85), bend your left knee and place the sole of your left foot against your right inner thigh. (If your lower back rounds, sit on a folded blanket.) Inhale and lengthen your spine; exhale and bend forward over your right leg as far as feels comfortable for your body. If you can, reach forward and hold onto the edges of your right foot with both hands. Draw your shoulders away from your ears as you press equally through the ball and heel of the right foot. (Switch sides to work the opposite part of the body.)

Benefits: Stretches the hamstrings and back muscles. Also stretches the inner thigh and lower back.

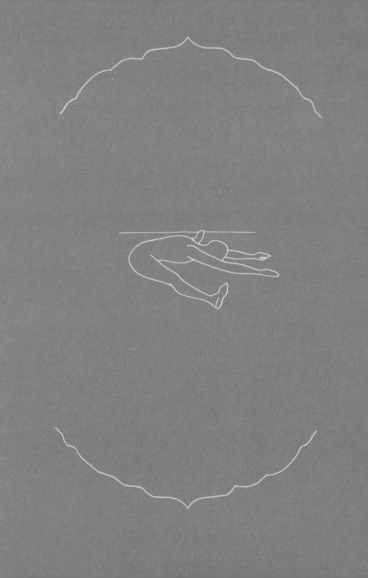

SEATED WIDE-LEGGED FORWARD BEND

UPAVISTHA KONASANA
(ooh-pah-VEE-stah cone-AH-sah-nah)

Origin: *Upavistha* means "seated," *kona* means "angle."

How to do it: From Staff Pose (page 85), lean back, placing your hands behind you, and open your legs wide apart. (If you need support, sit on a folded blanket.) Breathe deeply as you gently lean forward and bring your arms in front of you. Walk your hands forward, between your wide legs, going only as far as your body will comfortably allow.

Benefits: Stretches the hamstrings, inner legs, and spine. Opens the hips.

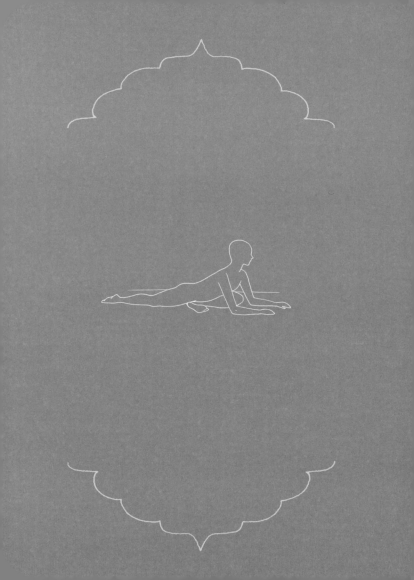

PIGEON POSE

Origin: With your chest lifted and your front leg tucked in like a wing, this pose is said to resemble a pigeon.

How to do it: From Downward-Facing Dog (page 55), bend your left knee in toward your chest, then turn the knee to the left and down toward the floor. Gently place your shin behind your left wrist. Adjust your left leg so it is positioned flat against the mat, with your knee pressing squarely into the mat. With your pelvis now square, place your fingertips on the floor in front of you. Breathe in, then exhale, and walk your hands forward as far as you can comfortably go, resting your forehead on the floor if you are able to take the pose deep enough. (Switch sides to work the opposite part of the body.)

Benefits: Opens the hips—front, inner, and outer.

Backbends

Backbends energize the body and open the heart while strengthening the spine, neck, and shoulders. They are also helpful in counteracting the effects of daily activities that constrict the chest, such as sitting, driving, and shallow breathing related to stress.

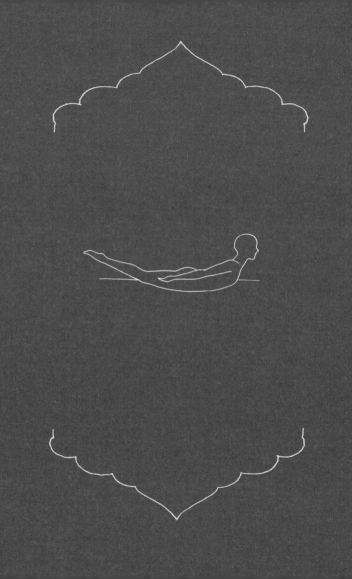

LOCUST POSE

SALABHASANA
(sha-lah-BAHS-ah-nah)

Origin: *Salabha* means "locust."

How to do it: Lie on your stomach with your forehead resting on the ground and your arms straight along your sides, palms facing the ground. Tuck your tailbone under slightly to reduce pressure on your lower back. Inhale, hug your inner thighs together, and lift your arms, legs, and head off the ground. Rather than trying to lift your body high, stretch it long instead, reaching your head and toes away from each other.

Benefits: Strengthens the entire back and the backs of the legs. Extends the spine, warming up the body for deeper backbends.

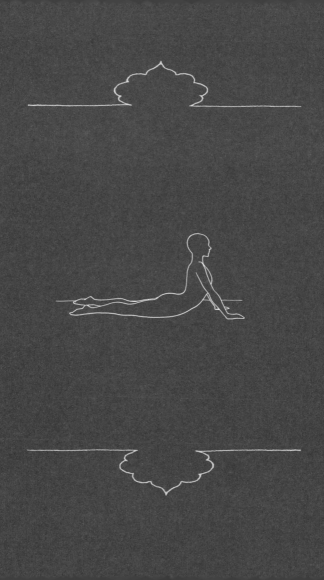

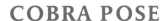

COBRA POSE

BHUJANGASANA
(boo-jahng-AH-sah-nah)

Origin: *Bhujanga* means "snake."

How to do it: Lie on your stomach, forehead resting
on the ground. Place your palms on the ground
underneath your shoulders. Hug your inner thighs
toward each other and press down through your
palms, gently lifting your head and upper chest off the
ground. Hug your elbows in alongside your rib cage
and straighten your arms as much as is comfortable
for you.

Benefits: Strengthens the arms, chest, and whole
back body. Prepares the body for deeper backbends by
warming up the spine.

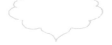

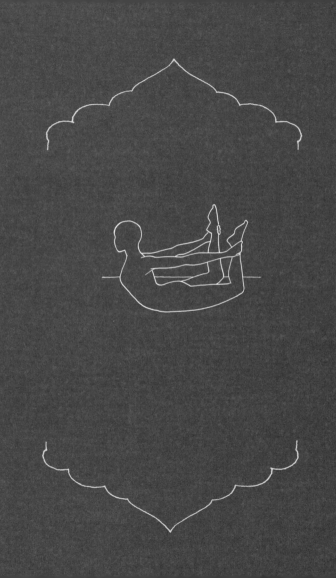

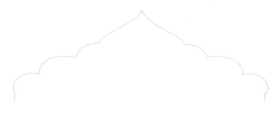

BOW POSE

DHANURASANA
(dahn-your-AHS-ah-nah)

Origin: *Dhanu* means "bow."

How to do it: Lie on your stomach with your forehead
resting on the ground. Bend both knees and reach
your arms back to grab your outer ankles. Inhale deeply
and then press your ankles back into your hands to lift
your head and chest off the ground. Slightly tuck your
tailbone under to keep your lower back long
and supported.

Benefits: Opens the chest, spine, and thighs.
Strengthens the back and hamstrings.

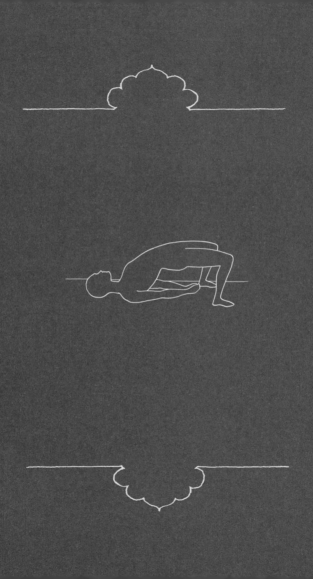

BRIDGE POSE

SETU BANDHA SARVANGASANA
(set-oo BAHN-dah sar-vahn-GAH-sah-nah)

Origin: *Setu* means "bridge."

How to do it: Lie on your back with your arms by your sides. Place both feet on the ground in line with your sitting bones, with your heels lightly touching your buttocks. Take a big breath in as you press down through your feet and lift your hips up, keeping your feet rooting into the mat. Clasp your hands together underneath your hips and shimmy your shoulders underneath you. Press down through your clasped hands to help you lift your hips higher.

Benefits: Strengthens the thighs, inner legs, and back. Opens the shoulders, spine, and chest.

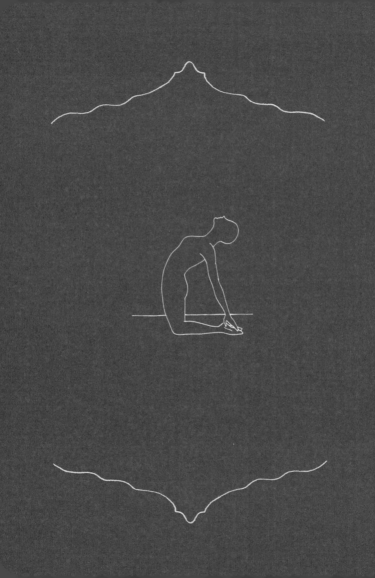

CAMEL POSE

USTRASANA
(oo-STRAS-ah-nah)

Origin: *Ustra* means "camel."

How to do it: Sit on your knees so your shins are parallel to each other and flat against the floor. Then lift your pelvis so that your hips are directly above your knees. Place your hands on your hips. As you inhale, lift your chest up and gently arch backward, going as far as your body will comfortably allow. If you are able to take it deeper, reach your arms behind you and touch your feet with your hands. Slightly tuck your tailbone under to keep your lower back long. Lift your heart and breathe.

Benefits: Stretches the whole front of the body—feet, thighs, abdomen, and chest. Stretches and strengthens the back.

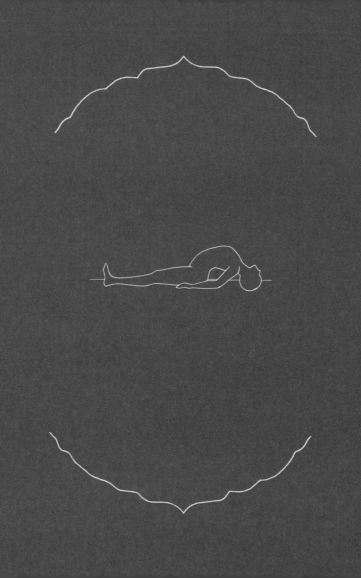

FISH POSE

MATSYASANA
(mats-YAS ah-nah)

Origin: *Matsya* means "fish."

How to do it: Lie on your back, with your upper body propped up by your elbows. Press your palms and forearms into the mat as you arch your chest, coming into a backbend. As you breathe into your chest, deepen the backbend. Slowly begin to move your chin away from your chest, mindfully allowing the crown of your head to come to the floor behind you. Squeeze your shoulder blades together and bring your shoulders away from your ears. Keep your legs active as you breathe.

Benefits: Opens the chest and neck.

Inversions

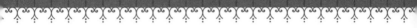

Inversions, which get your feet high above your head, are thought to be healing poses that stimulate your immune and endocrine systems, bringing fresh blood and nourishment to the brain and internal organs. By going upside down, you give your heart and mind a break—and see life from a new perspective.

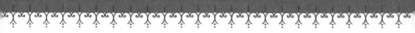

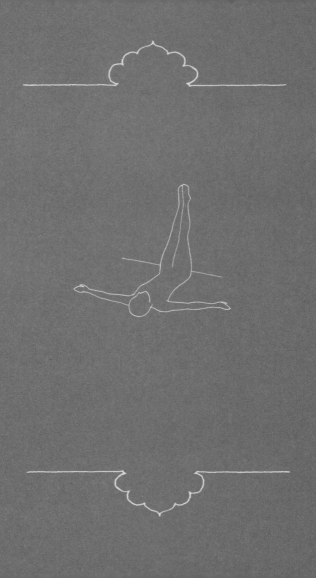

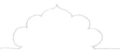

LEGS UP THE WALL

VIPARITA KARANI
(vi-pa-REE-ta ka-RON-ee)

Origin: *Viparita* means "inverted," *karani* means "action."

How to do it: Lie on your back parallel to a wall with your right hip alongside the wall. Then lift your legs, one at a time, so they sweep up the wall in a clockwise direction. Your body from the waist up will move across the floor until it is perpendicular to the wall. Keep your knees slightly bent. If there is a lot of space between your buttocks and the wall, bend your knees and scoot your buttocks closer to the wall. Slowly straighten your legs. Bring your arms out to the sides, palms facing up. Close your eyes and breathe deeply into your chest.

Benefits: Alleviates fatigue. Boosts circulation. Stretches the backs of the legs.

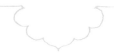

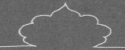

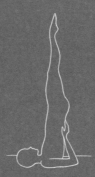

*Note: *Practice shoulder stand very carefully to avoid injury to the neck. Ask your teacher about ways you can protect yourself; for example, by placing a folded blanket under your shoulders to support your neck.*

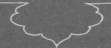

SHOULDER STAND

SARVANGASANA
(sar-van-GA-sah-nah)

Origin: *Salamba* means "support," *sarva* means "all,"
anga means "limb."

How to do it: Lie down and bring your arms alongside your
body and press your palms into the mat. Bend your knees and
bring them toward your head as your back lifts from the floor,
continuing to press your palms into the floor. Then bring your
palms to your lower back for support. Lift your pelvis over
your shoulders and straighten your legs so that they form an
extended vertical line with your torso. Walk your hands down
your back so your body rises higher, and bring your elbows
closer together, continuously working your body toward a
vertical position. Lift through your feet and firm your shoulder
blades on your back. Keep your head straight and avoid turning your head from side to side. Continue lifting, lengthening,
and breathing.

Benefits: Stretches the shoulders, neck, and throat.
Energizes the body. Promotes healthy digestion.

Resting Poses

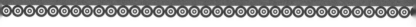

Resting poses promote calm and relaxation. Usually done at the end of class or throughout the class for periods of rest, they encourage the yogi to calm their breath, relax their mind, and reap the rewards of their practice.

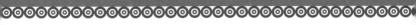

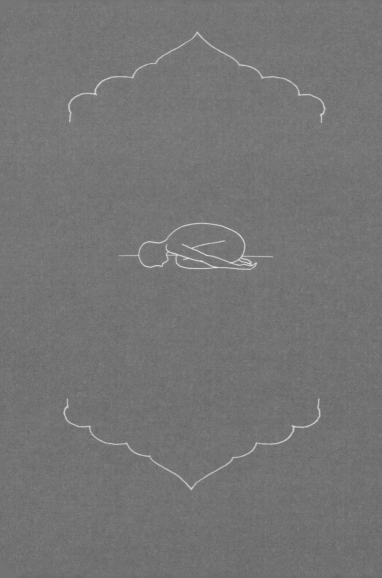

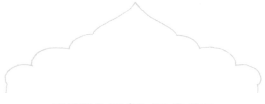

CHILD'S POSE

BALASANA
(bah-LAS-ah-nah)

Origin: *Bala* means "child."

How to do it: Kneel on your mat with your big toes touching behind you. Bring your knees hip-width apart, and slowly lower your torso down to the mat so it rests between your thighs and so that your head touches the floor. Bring your hands alongside your body and allow your shoulder blades to relax toward the floor.

Benefits: Stretches the ankles, hips, and thighs. Relieves lower back pain.

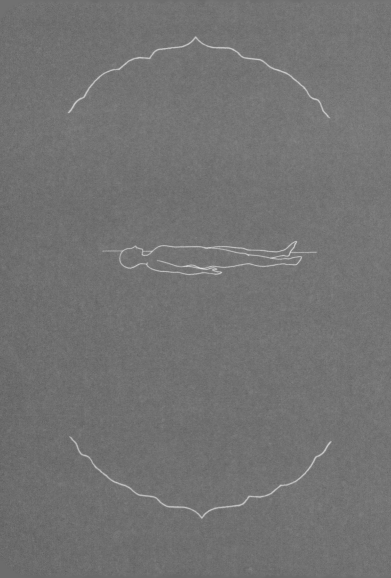

CORPSE POSE

SAVASANA
(sha-VAS-ah-nah)

Origin: *Sava* means "corpse."

How to do it: Lie flat on your back with your hands a few fist-widths away from your thighs, palms facing up. Spread your feet hip-width apart, and relax your toes. Then relax your jaw, tongue, and eyes. Wiggle your arms, hands, torso, legs, and feet, and then let them rest comfortably. Allow your body to sink into the floor. With each exhale, release any stress or tension from the day. Breathe deeply, focusing on the exhalations. Maintain a relaxed awareness, and let go of your troubles.

Benefits: Quiets the mind. Reduces fatigue. Promotes relaxation.

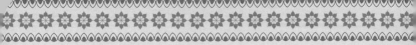

• *Namaste* and *Om* •

Namaste encapsulates the yoga tradition in one small but powerful word. Loosely translated as "The light in me greets the light in you," it is a recognition of each person's inner light, or divinity. Another well-known Sanskrit word, *Om*, is understood to signify everything—all of creation, all of consciousness. It's often chanted in unison at the beginning and end of a yoga class, where it might be pronounced as a long, drawn-out "aauuuoooooommm." *Om* is recognized as one of the world's most sacred *mantras* (see page 172). It is believed to bring the speaker closer to the vast interconnectedness of life.

• Yoga's Five Rules of Thumb •

Whatever style of yoga you choose to practice, or however inexperienced or skilled you may be, here are some basic rules to follow for safety and to get the most out of each session:

1. **Move gently.** As you move, imagine your body gliding through water. See how smoothly and rhythmically you can flow.

2. **Breathe easily.** Let your breath guide you. If you notice that you are gasping for air or holding your breath, this is a sure sign to ease up.

3. **Feel no pain.** Pain is your body's way of telling you you're going too far. Reach for your "edge"—that place where you feel perfectly challenged, where it's not too easy but not too hard. Only you can know your edge. Keep watch for your edge at all times, and take care not to risk injury by moving past it.

4. **No competition.** Yoga is a uniquely individual practice. It can be difficult to not compare yourself to others in a yoga class. Remember that every body has its own unique history and its own particular needs.

5. **Create a safe space.** Think of your yoga mat as a safe space to take a break from your perfectionist self, a place where you can accept and even love your perceived imperfections.

Part Three

Yoga Philosophy

The Eight-Limbed Path

Modern-day yoga is known for its physical poses, but the poses are just one step on what the ancient yogis believed was a path to enlightenment. The Eight-Limbed Path—outlined by prolific sage Patanjali (born between 300 BCE–AD 200) in his collection of writings called *The Yoga Sutra*—is a system of moral and ethical guidelines, and specific practices including yoga poses that lead the yogi to a peaceful life. Thousands of years after the Eight Limbs were first recorded, many yoga schools still use them as the foundation of their practice, while individual yogis find that they apply seamlessly to everyday living, off the mat.

The eight limbs of the Eight-Limbed Path—like the limbs of a tree—are integrally linked to each other, proceeding in a basic order, from external to internal, guiding us toward inner peace. Our journey starts with the first limb, or *yama,* which consists of five principles that help make us aware of how we see and interact with the external world. Next, we arrive at *niyama,* the second limb, which also consists of five principles. The *niyamas* invite us to look inward and truly get to know ourselves through reflection and self-study. The third and fourth limbs are active, energetic practices. In Patanjali's day, the third limb, or *asana*, meant a comfortable seated position. Today it refers to yoga's physical poses. The fourth limb, *pranayama*, meant a practice of slowing the breath, and has since evolved into the various breathing exercises that we know today. Both of these limbs, *asana* and *pranayama*, prepare the body and mind for the three limbs that follow: *pratyahara*, inward focus by withdrawing the five senses; *dharana*, concentration; and *dhyana*, meditation. The eighth and final limb—which is understood to be the ultimate reward—is *samadhi*, described by some as ecstasy and by others more simply as enlightenment, contentment, or inner peace.

Samadhi is a grandiose concept, but Patanjali and the ancient yogis believed it to be achievable by every human being of any means. Indeed, today we might understand *samadhi* to be the natural, blissful reward of being kind to others, nurturing the self, and living in the moment. The following pages provide overviews of each limb of the Eight-Limbed Path, and offer modern-day applications of this ancient wisdom.

THE EIGHT LIMBS

1. Yama: Universal morality (page 138)
2. Niyama: Personal morality (page 139)
3. Asana: Physical practices (page 140)
4. Pranayama: Breathing practices (page 141)
5. Pratyahara: Withdrawal of the senses (page 142)
6. Dharana: Concentration (page 143)
7. Dhyana: Meditation (page 144)
8. Samadhi: Enlightenment (page 145)

The Five Yamas

1. Ahimsa: Nonharming (page 147)
2. Satya: Honesty (page 148)
3. Asteya: Not stealing (page 149)
4. Brahmacharya: Sensual moderation (page 150)
5. Aparigraha: Nonpossessiveness (page 151)

The Five Niyamas

1. Saucha: Purity (page 153)
2. Santosha: Contentment (page 154)
3. Tapas: Self-discipline (page 155)
4. Svadhyaya: Self-study (page 156)
5. Ishvara pranidhana: Surrender (page 157)

1. Yama

UNIVERSAL MORALITY

The *yamas*, loosely translated from Sanskrit as "restraints," offer five ethical guidelines for behaviors to avoid in daily life. In this first limb of the Eight-Limbed Path, the focus is on the yogi's relations with the external world. By shifting how they view the external world and by making adjustments to how they interact with others, they prepare themselves for the internal self-improvement that lies ahead (see The Five Yamas, page 146).

In action: View the *yamas* as what *not* to do. Don't hurt others. Don't lie or steal. Don't misuse your sensuality or be greedy. Follow these simple rules, yoga wisdom says, and you'll reduce your suffering while increasing the happiness of others.

2. Niyama

PERSONAL MORALITY

Having improved their outlook and interactions with others by applying the *yamas*, the yogi turns inward and applies *niyama*, the second limb of the Eight-Limbed Path. The *niyamas*, loosely translated as "observances," are five guidelines that promote self-betterment, leading a step closer to the ultimate goal: Inner peace (see The Five Niyamas, page 152).

In action: Use the *niyamas* to support your personal, internal growth. Get to know yourself. Cleanse your mind, your home, and the environment. Cultivate contentment and discipline. Surrender attachments—to belongings, bad habits, and negative thoughts, for example.

3. Asana

PHYSICAL PRACTICES

Many today are surprised to learn that yoga's physical poses are only a small part of a traditional yoga practice. Originally, they were meant to prepare the mind and body for meditation—the seventh limb—which requires long periods of sitting. Yoga poses, called *asanas* (*asana* means "seat"), make the yogi strong, energetic, flexible, and calm, releasing long-held tensions in the body and opening it up to new possibilities.

In action: Engage your body by challenging yourself physically. Attend a yoga class, or lay out your mat in your home and cycle through some poses (see Yoga Poses, page 36). Set an intention: What do you want to gain? What do you want to lose? Make a commitment to that moment, and cultivate discipline by practicing daily, weekly, or as it suits you. And embrace the fact that, as a "practice," yoga is never complete or finished, but rather is an ongoing process—a journey that is the destination itself.

4. Pranayama
BREATHING PRACTICES

While the physical body is refined through yoga poses, the energetic body is refined through breathing practices, which encourage energy to flow freely throughout your body. *Prana* means "life force," and the breath is seen as a primary vehicle for transporting life force. *Ayama* means "control." *Pranayama* means aiding the movement of life force through the body by controlling the breath, and is a foundation of yoga practice. Focused breathing has both calming and energizing effects on the body and mind, key preparations for the steps ahead on the Eight-Limbed Path.

In action: Improve your breathing habits by simply taking note of them. Inhale. Exhale. At what point does your breath feel constricted? When do you get restless? Gain an awareness of your breath by exploring the breathing exercises in this book (see page 162).

5. Pratyahara

WITHDRAWAL OF THE SENSES

The fifth limb of the Eight-Limbed Path trains the yogi to overcome distractions such as fear, cravings, and desires, by withdrawing the five senses (sight, sound, smell, taste, and touch). By shifting the focus away from the outside world, you are able to more clearly observe yourself and gain powerful self-awareness.

In action: The next time you feel a craving, fear, or desire, use it as an opportunity to practice *pratyahara*. First, acknowledge the urge in a nonjudgmental way. Notice the thoughts and feelings related to it. How does your body feel? What is your mind telling you? How would it feel to give in? How would it feel to *not* give in? The self-knowledge that results from gentle observation of your thoughts and feelings can enable you to resist these distractions and focus instead on planting seeds of inner peace.

6. Dharana

CONCENTRATION

The sixth limb invites the yogi to apply their newly rewarded clear-headedness to a new goal: Concentration. By focusing attention on a single point, one can still the mind, further bolstering it against harmful distractions and preparing the yogi for the next step on the Eight-Limbed Path: Meditation.

In action: Whether you are preparing for meditation or just want to sharpen your focus, concentration is a valuable tool for staying in the present moment and offering your undivided attention to yourself, your hobbies or occupation, and your loved ones. Practice concentration by finding a comfortable seated position. Choose a word, phrase, object, or sound to focus on. Notice when you become distracted, and gently guide your attention back to your point of focus as often as needed.

7. Dhyana

MEDITATION

Meditation is an ancient practice that enables the mind to enter a state of uninterrupted concentration and relaxed calm. The previous six limbs of the Eight-Limbed Path have prepared the yogi for this step by slowly and intentionally guiding them inward, helping them detach from distracting external influences. Meditation, the seventh limb, delivers the yogi to the eighth and final limb, *samadhi*—a blissful state, free from suffering.

In action: Flex your new concentration skills with one of the meditation exercises in this book (see page 166). Be prepared for constant interruption, as thoughts and sensations will inevitably intrude on your focus. Don't judge yourself if you're not "good at it." Meditate, perhaps, on self-acceptance.

8. Samadhi

ENLIGHTENMENT

The eighth and final limb, *samadhi*, is the ultimate reward—a blissful state known by many names: ecstasy; enlightenment; inner peace; union with the divine; a feeling of oneness with the world; a sense that everyone and everything is connected; freedom; happiness. According to ancient tradition, *samadhi* is achieved at the height of meditation. In reality, it can be achieved any time the self is engaged intentionally, compassionately, and honestly.

In action: There are an infinite number of ways to experience *samadhi*, for no two people are alike. What's *your* version of *samadhi*? When do you get that feeling that all is right in the world? For some, *samadhi* happens in nature—in a forest or at the ocean's edge. For others, it happens when cooking a meal for loved ones, composing a poem, or playing with children. It might happen in short, fleeting flashes. Or it might linger just long enough for you to study its brilliance, challenging you to stay present in the moment while it lasts—not grasping at it, developing attachments, or fearing its departure. It might happen frequently or rarely, under good circumstances or bad, when you're alone or among crowds. *Samadhi* takes many shapes and forms and it's always within reach. In time, and with practice, you might come to see life—in all its glorious imperfection—as *samadhi* itself.

The Five Yamas

Yama is the first limb of yoga's Eight-Limbed Path. Also translated as "restraints," the *yamas* introduce five ethical guidelines that focus on the ways of viewing the external world and interacting with others. The *yamas*, such as telling the truth and not stealing, are considered a foundation of a yoga practice.

THE FIVE YAMAS

1. Ahimsa: Nonharming

2. Satya: Honesty

3. Asteya: Not stealing

4. Brahmacharya: Sensual moderation

5. Aparigraha: Nonpossessiveness

1. Ahimsa

NONHARMING

Not harming others—or *ahimsa*, a nonharming mindset—is the ultimate starting point on the yogi's path to peaceful living. Living a life of nonviolence means not indulging in physical, verbal, or emotional abuse of others, or yourself. Self-abuse includes holding one's self to unrealistic ideals and striving for perfection. Also loosely translated as "compassion," *ahimsa* means adopting a kind, forgiving, and gentle approach to life.

In action: Sit quietly observing your thoughts, and notice when an unkind thought about another person— or a thought that's unkind to yourself—arises. Hold that thought in your mind, and release it with an exhale. Then, think the opposite thought (even if you might not believe it). Try this a few times throughout the day, creating new positive thought patterns to replace the old, negative ones. After you've practiced this on your own, try it when you are with others. When you notice tensions are mounting, release negative thoughts with an exhale.

2. Satya
HONESTY

Telling the truth is more than simply not lying. Real honesty goes far beyond words. *Satya*, the yogic practice of honesty, requires the yogi to study themselves closely and own up to limitations that can lead to dishonest behavior. It requires one to acknowledge how they might differ from the person others think them to be, and to correct misconceptions, despite the discomfort that often goes along with being truthful. It sometimes requires one to say "no" despite the pressure to say "yes."

In action: Observe yourself the next time someone says something that upsets you. First, notice your immediate reaction. Do you ignore them just to smooth things over? Do you defensively interject? Do you reply passive-aggressively? Ask yourself how you *really* feel, and recognize how difficult it is to be straightforward and honest. In that moment, summon the honest reaction that's in harmony with your inner truth.

3. Asteya
NOT STEALING

Asteya, or nonstealing, means more than simply not taking something that belongs to someone else. For at the root of stealing is dissatisfaction with one's own belongings or circumstances. This dissatisfaction manifests itself in numerous unhealthy behaviors—not just stealing but also comparing one's self to others, and indulging in that insatiable human need for more, more, more. Dissatisfaction is a true obstacle on the yogi's path to enlightenment. The antidote is gratitude. Practicing *asteya* guides the yogi to recognize what they *do* have, which nourishes self-acceptance and a more clear-eyed, compassionate view of others.

In action: When you feel that old familiar sense of dissatisfaction creeping in, take a moment to identify the root cause. What left you feeling like you have less than enough? What are you craving or longing for, and why? Now turn inward and take inventory of your strengths and blessings. Accept your circumstances, and you'll discover a peace that can't be found anywhere but inside yourself.

4. Brahmacharya

SENSUAL MODERATION

The ancient practice of *brahmacharya* involved the yogi taking a vow of celibacy. It was believed that sensual desires and related actions required too much energy—energy that was better invested in one's spiritual awakening. Today's yogis take a broader view of this guideline, seeing it as an opportunity to practice moderation. It urges one to avoid addiction; to be thoughtful about how one indulges the five senses; and to reflect on the intention's outcomes (good and bad) with the aim of boosting the honesty and integrity of one's actions.

In action: You don't need to be celibate to be a yogi. But you might consider how you can make your self-indulgences more of an expression of your own divine nature. On an even broader level, simply consider where your energy is going each day. When might it be wasted, and how can you channel more of it toward your search for inner peace?

5. Aparigraha

NONPOSSESSIVENESS

A practice of *aparigraha* encourages the yogi to let go of attachments. It acknowledges the human need to collect things—material possessions, emotions, accomplishments—in order to feel safe, wealthy, entertained, and valuable to others. Letting go welcomes in a basic faith that the universe will provide, and frees one from the clinging and worry that accompany attachment, creating room in one's life for fresh possibilities and powerful positive energy.

In action: Consider giving something away. Not that unwanted item you've never used, but something you truly love. Have faith that something even more meaningful will arrive to take its place. Now look at an emotion—a fear, hope, or resentment. Consider how it's tying you down, and how it might own you, rather than the other way around. Move on to new discoveries and feel the lightness and freedom that come with letting go, one attachment at a time.

The Five Niyamas

Translated as "observances," the *niyamas* are the second limb of Patanjali's Eight-Limbed Path. While the first limb, the *yamas*, addresses the external world and how one relates to others, the *niyamas* deal with the inner world—personal rather than interpersonal guidelines.

THE FIVE NIYAMAS

1. Saucha: Purity
2. Santosha: Contentment
3. Tapas: Self-discipline
4. Svadhyaya: Self-study
5. Ishvara pranidhana: Surrender

1. Saucha

PURITY

Purity, according to ancient yoga tradition, is attained by cleansing the mind and body. Loosely interpreted, it extends to any aspect of the yogi's life—personal hygiene, home, thoughts, or the environment at large. The aim is to create and maintain pure energy inside and out, and to clear the literal and figurative path to enlightenment.

In action: Reflect on the areas of your life where clutter has collected. Your body? Try a three-day diet cleanse, eating only grains and vegetables and drinking plenty of water. Your environment? Clean out your closets and unload those possessions that are holding you back. Your attention span? Take a media fast in which you turn off your computer and phone for an hour, a day, or a weekend. Your spirituality? Create your own cleansing ritual; for example, write down emotions you'd like to release, then burn the list in a campfire. Enjoy the rewards of pure, fresh energy rejuvenating your soul and your surroundings.

2. Santosha

CONTENTMENT

A practice of *santosha* guides the yogi to be content with their circumstances, no matter what they are. Not quite as easy as it sounds, cultivating contentment means resisting self-doubt, curbing jealousy, and recognizing that there is not just one way to happiness, but a unique path for every human being. Actively accepting what one already has—the good and the bad—and bolstering the self against changing circumstances is the essence of *santosha*.

In action: The next time things don't turn out as you hoped, take a moment to consider the many different ways you can choose to react. Consider, too, that you can choose *not* to react. Not reacting can signify that you accept what is happening, without fear, judgment, or expectation. With practice, the quality of your contentment will deepen, as you are reassured, time and again, that your contentment holds strong despite the ever-changing circumstances around you.

3. Tapas

SELF-DISCIPLINE

Tapas means "heat" or "burn," signifying the intense commitment required to bring about transformation in the same way that metal is shaped by fire. *Tapas* is often called upon in times of crisis when extra endurance or commitment is required. The wise yogi stokes their inner fire any number of times throughout the day; for example, when they feel they are faltering in their commitment to self-betterment, when they are holding a difficult yoga pose for an especially long time, and when they are struggling to resist temptation—or facing any other obstacle on their quest for enlightenment.

In action: The next time you're struggling to hold a yoga pose—when your thigh gets wobbly in Extended Side Angle Pose, for example, or when your mind wanders—envision the glowing coals inside you, and persevere. *Tapas* will energize and enable you to act with integrity and intention. *Tapas* is what gives you the energy to push through challenges and difficulties, knowing that when you do, the rewards on the other side will be worth it. Apply perseverance to your daily life while cultivating self-reliance and faith that any situation can be endured and any circumstance overcome.

4. Svadhyaya

SELF-STUDY

Svadhyaya, the yogic practice of self-study, traditionally meant engrossing one's self in texts and scriptures. Today's yogi practices self-study in a different way, but with the same goals in mind: to tap into the true self, to make decisions that are better aligned with one's individual callings, and, in doing so, to live a more authentic life.

In action: Get to know yourself. One way to practice self-study is by keeping a journal. Record the events of your day or thoughts that might provide you with a window into your soul. Be honest with yourself as you write, consciously clearing away the superficialities that obscure who you really are. Over time, as you look back through its pages, you'll come to recognize patterns in your thinking and behavior, both good and bad. Self-knowledge facilitates growth and plants seeds of wisdom and inner peace.

5. Ishvara pranidhana
SURRENDER

Ishvara pranidhana loosely translates to "surrender to the supreme being." Yoga, considered to be a non-religious practice, invites the yogi to interpret their own meaning of divinity. Whatever it may mean, and wherever it might be found—in nature, among friends and family, or in the present moment—the yogi is encouraged to surrender to it. This might mean releasing attachments to outcomes, releasing one's self from judgments and expectations, having faith in something outside the self, and liberating the self from the grip of the ego.

In action: Welcome each day with a *mantra*, and repeat it when you feel the familiar pull of attachments: *Let go. Let go. Let go.*

Part Four

Beyond the Poses

Yoga isn't just physical poses; it's a comprehensive system that incorporates many other practices that can transform. Each of the following tools and techniques—breathing, meditation, *mantras*, *mudras*, *bandhas*, and *chakras*—represents an opportunity to support and deepen one's yoga practice. For example, chanting a mantra at the beginning of a yoga session can help set one's intention. During the session, activating the *chakras* can bring the focus to certain areas of the body. And after the session, the body is calm and the mind is clear—both well prepped for meditation.

Outside of class, and independent of the poses, these tools and techniques can be equally effective at restoring balance. Breathing exercises, for example, can provide an energy boost any time of day, while meditation can be adapted for any environment. Moving beyond the poses presents an opportunity for transformation and growth. Building on the foundation of physical poses, these techniques help a yoga practice strengthen and blossom over time.

Breathing

Yogis believe that breath is the link between the body and the mind. In yoga, the practice of breathing is called *pranayama*, the control of *prana*, or life force. *Pranayama*, the fourth limb of the Eight-Limbed Path (see page 134), takes the yogi one step closer to enlightenment by helping to control and direct the body's energy through breathing exercises. The following three exercises offer a sampling of traditional techniques and healthful benefits in a breathing practice.

COOLING BREATH

Sanskrit name: *Sitali*

Pronunciation: sit-AL-ee

Benefit: Calming

In the yoga tradition, anger, frustration, and anxiety are associated with too much heat in the body. This cooling breath helps to get rid of some of the body's heat and help restore a sense of balance and concentration.

How to do it: Bring the tip of the tongue slightly outside your mouth and fold your tongue lengthwise into a tube shape. Slightly lower your chin. Inhale, drawing in air through the tube (creating a hissing sound). Your neck should be comfortable, not strained. Fill the lungs. Then bring your tongue in, close the mouth, and exhale slowly through the nose. Repeat.

DEEP ABDOMINAL BREATHING

Sanskrit name: *Dirga Swasam*

Pronunciation: DEER-ga swha-SAHM

Benefit: Relaxing

This simple breathing technique—also referred to as a "three-part breath" because of how air is directed into three areas of the lungs: the abdomen, diaphragm, and chest—is an excellent counteragent to the choppy, shallow breathing we resort to during the average stressful day. Deep abdominal breathing can slow down the heart rate, rid the body of stale air, and activate the energetic pathways in the body. Perhaps even more impactful, it can stimulate the parasympathetic nervous system, which sends instant calm throughout the body.

How to do it: Find a comfortable position, seated or lying down. Bring one hand to your belly. As you inhale through your nose, feel your abdomen rise. As you exhale through your nose, pull it slightly in so the navel draws toward the spine. With each inhalation, fill your abdomen, diaphragm, and chest with air, all the way to the tops of your ribs. With each exhalation, empty the air from your lungs completely and draw the navel slightly in. Leave your hand on your abdomen as a guide to this three-part breath, and continue the exercise for five minutes.

ALTERNATE NOSTRIL BREATHING

Sanskrit name: *Nadi Shodhana*

Pronunciation: NAD-ee SHOW-donna

Benefit: Balancing

This breathing technique is thought to balance your energy by balancing the right and left hemispheres of your brain.

How to do it: Find a comfortable seated position. Start to breathe regularly. Bring your right hand to your nose, with your thumb near the right nostril and your fourth and fifth fingers near your left nostril. Take a complete exhalation through both nostrils. Close off the right nostril with your thumb and inhale slowly through the left. At the top of the inhalation, close off the left side with your left fingers, release the thumb from the right side, and exhale slowly out through the right nostril. Then inhale through the right, then close off the right as you release the left, and exhale. Continue with this pattern—inhale, switch; exhale, inhale, switch; exhale, inhale, switch—for three minutes.

Meditation

Meditation is an ancient practice that develops a sense of calm, peace, and serenity. It brings one back to the present moment, and it develops what is called the "witness"—the ability to observe oneself, without getting caught up in emotions.

Meditation and yoga poses are intrinsically tied together. Both are key steps on the yogi's path to enlightenment, or the Eight-Limbed Path (see page 134). Historically, yoga's physical poses were done to prepare the body for meditation, relaxing, and opening the body to enable the yogi to sit comfortably for long periods of time without discomfort. Today, meditation is a wonderful way to deal with the stresses of modern life by taking the time to stop and become one with the present moment.

How to Meditate: the Basics

Imagine a beautiful, smooth lake. Now picture a stone skipping across that lake, causing the water to ripple. Your mind is that lake. Your thoughts are the stones that agitate the surface. When you learn to meditate, you learn to keep your mind clear and the lake smooth, even when thoughts, emotions, and circumstances threaten to interfere.

Start a meditation session by sitting still, breathing deeply, and focusing the mind. Thoughts will arise. You are hungry, thirsty, tired, annoyed. So be it. Your mind wanders. Allow it. The idea isn't to banish all thoughts but just to notice them. See those thoughts as separate from yourself. "Witness" them with a neutral, nonjudgmental mindset. Over time, your focus will improve. You'll let go more easily. You'll acquire meditation skills that can be applied in any setting. Begin by trying one of the meditation techniques ahead: Mindfulness Meditation, Compassion Meditation, and Walking Meditation.

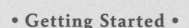

• Getting Started •

Meditation Tips

- Find a quiet spot where you feel peaceful and won't be disturbed.
- The traditional time to meditate is morning, because it's a quiet time of renewal.
- Start out meditating for five minutes each day for a week, and increase the time each week by five minutes.
- Set up a timer so you don't keep checking the clock.
- When you feel drowsy or distracted, continue bringing your awareness back to your breath.

Meditation Positions

- **Cross-legged.** Sit in a cross-legged position and rock your pelvis back and forth a few times to find a position where your lower back has a slight natural, inward curve. If your back is rounded, sit on a pillow, cushion, or folded-up towel.
- **Legs outstretched.** Sit on the floor with your legs stretched out in front of you. Rock from side to side until your sitting bones are connecting with the floor. If your lower back is rounded in this position and not perfectly upright, sit on a pillow, cushion, or folded-up towel.
- **Seated in a chair.** Bring the soles of your feet to the floor, and allow them to ground you. Imagine that a string is attached to the top of your head and someone is gently pulling on it, lengthening the back of your neck and your spine.
- **Kneeling.** Sit on the tops of your feet, or put a pillow underneath your buttocks.

MINDFULNESS MEDITATION

Mindfulness meditation involves noticing your thoughts, identifying and labeling them, and then releasing them without allowing them to take root. To be mindful is simply to be aware; and to label and then release is to let go. Being mindful and letting go are two foundations of the yoga mindset, and are simple practices that can be applied throughout the day to stay calm and present.

Technique: Find a comfortable position. Feel the sensations in your body. Then start to notice your thoughts and feelings. As thoughts wander into your mind, start to label them: *Planning. Worrying. Thinking.* Then let them go. It's natural for the mind to wander, so try to resist becoming frustrated when it does. Simply return to the task at hand: noticing, labeling, and letting go. Throughout, focus on your breath.

COMPASSION MEDITATION

Compassion meditation is a wonderful way to bring peace to yourself and others. It's a meaningful exercise in acknowledging your connections to all people, that we are all equals, and that we are all part of the same whole.

Technique: Start by sitting in a comfortable position. Breathe gently in and out. When you feel ready, silently repeat the words *May I be safe. May I be happy. May I be healthy. May I live with ease.* Gently repeat these phrases in your mind. (If you have other wishes, make substitutions.) Next, think of a friend or loved one. With them in your mind and heart, repeat *May you be safe. May you be happy. May you be healthy. May you live with ease.* Then think of a neutral person in your life—a neighbor, your bus driver, the person behind the cash register—and repeat the phrases with them in mind. Next think of someone with whom you are engaged in conflict. Repeat the same words, picturing them in your mind. Finally, imagine the whole universe in your mind, and meditate: *May all beings live in safety, be happy, be healthy, live with ease.*

WALKING MEDITATION

Walking meditation symbolizes the yogic belief that the journey is more important than the destination. It trains the yogi to pay attention to their movements, surroundings, and experience while resisting other thoughts or concerns that may threaten to intrude.

Technique: Stand in a comfortable position, ideally outdoors. Begin to walk slowly, noticing each micromovement of your body. After a few minutes, slow down your pace and concentrate on each step. Notice how the sole of your foot connects to the ground with each step. When your mind wanders, stay present and aware of the experience and any sensations in your body. Scan your body for any tension; and when you discover it, actively release that part of your body. Keep your gaze calm and steady, and your breath even, and continue keeping your focus on the activity and bodily sensations of walking.

Mantras

The Sanskrit word *mantra* loosely translates as "divine speech" or transformative sound. A well-known example is "*Om*" (see page 130), which is often chanted at the beginning and end of a yoga class. Like a prayer that is sung, a mantra can have calming, healing, and meditative benefits. According to yoga tradition, sound creates a physical vibration in the body, which clears the *chakras* (see page 180) and makes the yogi feel more peaceful and alive. Here are a few beloved, classic mantras.

OM SHANTI

Pronunciation: oooom SHAN-tee

Translation: *Om* reflects the whole world, *shanti* means peace.

What it means: This simple mantra is a prayer for peace within yourself, and within all beings.

OM MANI PADME HUM

Pronunciation: om MAN-ee PAD-may om

Translation: "The jewel in the lotus of the heart"

What it means: This popular mantra refers to the hidden spark of divinity within each human being. Inspired by the lotus flower that takes root in the mud yet blossoms beautifully toward the sun, it offers a reminder that transformation is possible under any circumstance.

OM NAMAH SHIVAYA

Pronunciation: om nah-mah shee-VAY ah

Translation: "I bow to the goodness within myself."

What it means: This beloved chant—often heard in today's yoga classrooms— has roots in the Hindu religion. It honors the god Shiva, who represents the goodness that exists within all things.

Mudras

Yoga's hand *mudras* are hand positions that can be incorporated into yoga sequences, breathing exercises, and a meditation practice. Hands and fingers are positioned to seal energy inside the body, helping its circulation. (The commonly accepted translation for the Sanskrit word *mudra* is "seal.") During a yoga session, *mudras* can signify strength, connection, or compassion. During a meditation session, they can bring calm, awareness, and focus to your body and mind. Three of the most common *mudras* are *Anjali mudra*, *Dhyana mudra*, and *Chin mudra*.

Anjali Mudra

This *mudra* is a gesture of honor and devotion. (The Sanskrit word *anjali* loosely translates to "offering.") Bringing the hands together in this way also symbolizes union, the definition of yoga. When done, it's thought to quiet your mind and open your heart.

How to do it: Bring the palms of your hands together, pressing your thumbs slightly into your sternum.

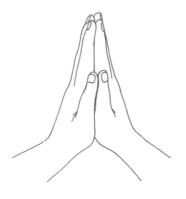

Dhyana mudra

A common *mudra* for seated meditation, this hand position is thought to bring a sense of peace and serenity to the mind. Some believe the triangle formed by the hands represents fire that burns out impurities.

How to do it: Bring your hands to your navel or lap. Place the right palm over the left and bring the tips of the thumbs together.

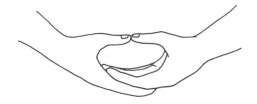

Chin Mudra

The index finger represents the small self (or the individual), while the thumb represents the big self (or the divine). Connecting them symbolizes union and allows energy to flow freely between the two, stimulating wisdom and knowledge. (*Chin* is loosely translated from Sanskrit to "consciousness" or "self-knowledge.")

How to do it: Either kneeling or sitting in a cross-legged position, bring your hands to your knees with the palms facing up. Join the tips of each thumb and index finger, leaving the other fingers extended and facing up.

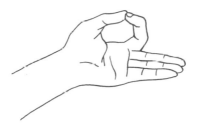

Bandhas

Bandhas are internal body locks that are activated by the contraction of muscle groups. They are thought to help the yogi regulate energy movement around the body while physically supporting the body in a yoga pose and helping to focus the mind. The following presents a very simplified overview of three commonly known *bandhas*. *Bandhas* are potentially powerful, so consult an experienced teacher before furthering your exploration.

MULA BANDHA

Pronunciation: MOO-la BAN-da

Also known as: root lock

Simplified version: As you exhale, gently contract the muscles in your pelvic floor. Imagine energy being blocked from exiting through the posterior of your body, and rising upward to support and stabilize you.

UDDIYANA BANDHA

Pronunciation: OO-dee-YAH-na-BAN-da

Also known as: abdominal lock

Simplified version: Gently contract your abdominal muscles toward your back as you complete an exhalation, and imagine your body's energy rising upward.

JALANDHARA BANDHA

Pronunciation: JA-lan-DA-ra BAN-da

Also known as: throat lock

Simplified version: After an exhalation, gently bring your chin toward your sternum while lengthening the back of the neck, imagining that precious energy is pooling at the top of the spine.

Chakras

According to ancient tradition, an underlying energetic structure exists within the physical structure of our skeleton and muscles. The *chakras* are thought to be energy centers of the body, envisioned as wheels with energy coiled inside them. (*Chakra* is a Sanskrit word loosely translated as "wheel.") Yoga poses, breathing practices, and mantras are believed to activate pathways called *nadis*, or energy channels. Activation brings *prana*, or life force, to the body's cells while also freeing stuck energy and cleansing the body.

There are seven *chakras*. The first is located at the base of the spine, and the seventh is located at the crown of the head. Most are linked to an element which is thought to play a role in balancing that *chakra*; and certain benefits or qualities of life can be enjoyed by balancing each *chakra*. Specific yoga poses are thought to be beneficial in balancing these energy centers.

THE SYMBOLS

The *chakras* are symbolized by the lotus flower. Each *chakra* symbol is a different color and has a different number of petals, and each includes a geometric design that represents the energies within that *chakra*. A small dot toward the center of the design, called a *bindu*, represents the True Self.

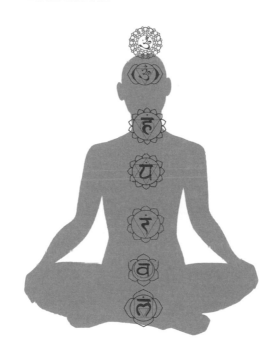

First Chakra

Sanskrit name: *Muladhara*

Also known as: Root *chakra*

Where it is: Base of the spine

Corresponding element: Earth

Corresponding benefit: Groundedness

Corresponding pose: Standing Forward
Bend (see page 45)

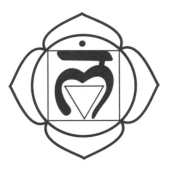

Second Chakra

Sanskrit name: *Svadhisthana*

Also known as: Sacral *chakra*

Where it is: Lower abdomen

Corresponding element: Water

Corresponding benefit: Pleasure

Corresponding pose: Seated Wide-Legged Forward Bend (see page 101)

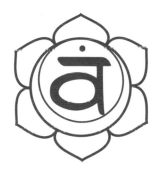

Third Chakra

Sanskrit name: *Manipura*

Also known as: Navel *chakra*

Where it is: Upper abdomen

Corresponding element: Fire

Corresponding benefit: Confidence

Corresponding pose: Full Boat Pose (see page 93)

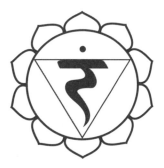

Fourth Chakra

Sanskrit name: *Anahata*

Also known as: Heart *chakra*

Where it is: Center of the chest

Corresponding element: Air

Corresponding benefit: Love

Corresponding pose: Cow-Face Pose (see page 89)

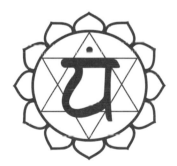

Fifth Chakra

Sanskrit name: *Visuddha*

Also known as: Throat *chakra*

Where it is: Throat

Corresponding element: Ether

Corresponding benefit: Communication

Corresponding pose: Bridge Pose (see page 113)

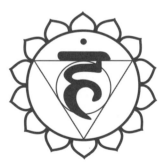

Sixth Chakra

Sanskrit name: *Ajna*

Also known as: Third-eye *chakra*

Where it is: Between the eyebrows

Corresponding element: None

Corresponding benefit: Intuition, wisdom

Corresponding pose: Child's Pose (see page 127)

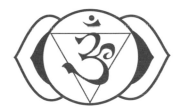

Seventh Chakra

Sanskrit name: *Sahasrara*

Also known as: Crown *chakra*

Where it is: Top of the head

Corresponding element: Thought

Corresponding benefit: Connection

Corresponding practice: Meditation (see page 166)

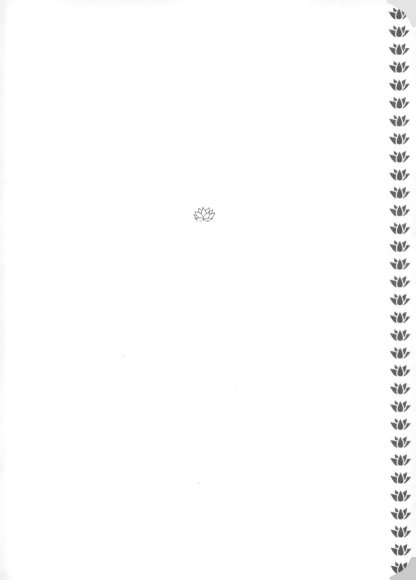

Part Five

Yoga Off the Mat

The perfect antidote to the stresses of modern life, yoga has a way of grounding us while at the same time setting us free. After just a few sessions with a skilled professional, your body will begin to grasp the basics, like a budding flower that naturally knows what to do in the sun. You'll leave class with steady breathing and a relaxed spine. And as you re-enter the day, you might slide your shoulder blades down your back and lift your heart to the sky, adapting the graceful movements you just performed on your mat to the "real world."

In time, your regular yoga practice might evolve into a lifestyle of peace and gratitude. You'll stand up a little taller. Breathe more deeply. Be more honest with yourself and others. When you lean down to pick something up, you might make your way into Forward Bend and linger there luxuriously for a moment. When reaching for something high on a shelf, you might kick a foot out behind you and find yourself in Dancer's Pose. When waiting for the bus on a crowded city street, you might transport yourself to a quiet forest with an improvised Tree Pose. You might offer friends or strangers an unspoken *Namaste* as you weave in and out of the day's encounters.

Nurture this evolution by actively bringing yoga off the mat and into your everyday life. The following tips offer ways to apply a physical yoga practice and mindset to the real world—upon waking and going to sleep, at school or at the office, on the road or in the air, and in relationships. No matter where you are, may your mat always await you in your mind, and may yoga's teachings guide you to peace and balance, inside and out.

Yoga at Work and School

Sitting all day at a computer can wreak havoc on your body, leaving you hunched over with neck pain or back aches. Let yoga come to your rescue—even if you can't fit a rolled-out yoga mat by your desk.

HALF DOG

Stand facing the back of your desk chair, about an arm's length away. (Make sure it's a sturdy, bottom-heavy chair that won't topple under your weight.) Bring your hands to the top of the chair, and lower your torso so that it's parallel with the floor; adjust your feet if needed. As you take a few deep breaths, feel the sides of your body lengthening, and the breath moving deeply into the back of your ribs. Stay here for a minute, and then get back to work.

FOREARM STRETCH

Stretch out your forearms and bring your palms together in front of your heart with your elbows out to the side. Slowly, bring your forearms toward each other. If you can, bring both elbows together as your fingertips rise toward the sky. Breathe deeply into the area between the shoulder blades, and relax your shoulders away from your ears.

SEATED TWIST

Bring your feet to the floor. Inhale and twist your torso to the left, bringing your right hand to your left thigh or left side of your chair. On each inhalation, lift your spine. On each exhalation, twist a little further. Come back to center, and repeat on the right side.

Yoga in Transit

Time spent traveling from point A to point B doesn't have to be stressful. It can be an ideal time to stretch the body and mind, despite the cramped space. Here are some tips for yogis on the move.

Air Travel

The small seats, minimal leg room, and long hours of sitting that go along with air travel can leave you literally bent out of shape. To avoid feeling bloated, achy, and cranky upon arrival, try these in-flight yoga poses—but be mindful of your neighbor.

SQUARE POSE

While seated, bring your left ankle up on top of your right knee. As you inhale, relax the left knee toward the floor while lengthening the spine. Keep the left foot flexed. As you exhale, lean slightly forward without rounding your back. Stay here for ten breaths, and repeat on the other side.

ARMS OVERHEAD

Interlace the fingers of your right hand with the fingers of your left hand, and bring your arms overhead, palms facing upward. Lengthen the sides of your body, press your palms toward the sky, and feel your shoulder blades move down your back. For a nice neck stretch, bring your chin toward your chest. Take a few deep breaths, then release. Readjust the interlacing of the hands and repeat the exercise.

SPINAL ROLLS

Sit up tall in your seat, then bend at the waist as far as you can, bringing your hands toward the floor. On an exhalation, tuck your tailbone under and slowly roll to an upright position, one vertebra at a time. When you come to a fully seated position, open your chest and roll your shoulders back and down. Take three deep breaths into your abdomen.

On the Road

Ground travel can be relaxing, but too much of it can take its toll on your body and mind. Car seats generally require one to sit with a tucked pelvis and a rounded spine, which can weaken posture over long periods of time. The stresses of the road—traffic jams and road rage, among others—can make it difficult for us to summon our compassion. Counter the effects by incorporating some yoga into your commutes and road trips. (These practices are suggested for passengers, not drivers.)

PELVIC TILTS

Rock your hips toward the front of your seat so that your lower back rounds. Then rock your hips toward the back of your seat so your lower back arches. Continue with alternating forward and backward movements. Link the movements to your breath—inhale forward, exhale backward—for gentle back relief.

SHOULDERS TO EARS

Lift your shoulders toward your ears, tensing your shoulder blades as you take three deep breaths. On an exhalation, release the shoulders with an audible sigh. Repeat three times for a quick pick-me-up.

BREATH AWARENESS

Throughout your trip, stay aware of your breath. Take full, deep breaths to bring *prana*, or energy, into the body. Focus on the back of your ribs. Start to breathe into the back ribs, feeling them fill up completely, and then exhale. Try inhaling as you count to one and exhaling as you count to two, which is known as the "1:2 breath." Complete five rounds and repeat, as needed.

Yoga in Relationships

Relationships can be more challenging than the most advanced yoga poses. No matter who is on the other end of a conflict—a friend, family member, coworker, schoolmate, or colleague—you can diffuse many situations by applying a yoga mindset and a few simple techniques.

BREATHE

When you are on the verge of saying something you will later regret, stop and take a few deep breaths. As you inhale, fill your abdomen with breath. As you exhale, release the air completely, and as you do so, imagine letting go of any anger and resentment. As you inhale, imagine drawing in compassion and kindness. Continue breathing until the impulsive urge passes.

MEDITATE

When faced with an important decision and in need of a clear-headed perspective, empty your mind with a brief meditation and then reconsider the decision. First, find a time and place where you won't be interrupted. Either lie down or be seated, and start to breathe. Notice any feelings that arise and gently acknowledge them without forcing them away. Once you have quieted the mind, imagine yourself in various scenarios related to the decision at hand. See each situation in your mind's eye, and notice how your body feels in that moment. Do you tense up? Feel relaxed? As your intuition speaks to you, take note, and resolve to tap into it when you have returned to your decision-making.

PRACTICE COMPASSION

It's easy to see the person on the other end of a conflict as "wrong" or "the enemy." But as yoga teaches us, we are all connected, and all equal. When judgments creep in, try repeating this classic mantra of compassion: *May you be safe. May you be happy. May you be healthy. May you live with ease.* (See page 170 for a related meditation practice.)

Yoga at Rest

Yoga can be just the thing you need to get your blood flowing and your mind calm before you start your day. And after a long day, yoga is a great way to unwind and get your mind and body ready for a good night's sleep.

Upon Waking

KNEES TO CHEST

Enjoy a full-body stretch, then bring your knees to your chest and wrap your arms around them. Slowly begin to draw small circles with the knees, first to the left and then to the right. Notice how this wakes up your spine. Try coordinating your breath with the movements.

LYING DOWN TWIST

Hug your knees to your chest and bring your arms out wide so they rest on the bed, creating a T-shape with the body. Slowly send your knees to the right, twisting the spine as you look toward your left hand. Engaging your abdominal muscles, inhale as you bring the knees back to center and repeat on the other side.

SINGLE-LEG HAMSTRING STRETCH

Straighten both legs. Extend the left leg up toward the ceiling, bringing your hands up to support the leg, holding anywhere except behind the knee. Keep the right leg engaged as you gently pull the left leg closer toward your body. After a few breaths, release the leg and repeat on the other side.

Before Bed

RELAXING EYE ROLLS

Give your eyes a rest with strain-releasing eye movements. Sit in a comfortable position on your bed, and close your eyes. Open your eyes and roll your eyeballs upward, as far as they can comfortably go. Then roll them down as far as they can comfortably go. Repeat three times, slowly, then close your eyes to rest for one breath. Next, open your eyes and move them to the left and right, as far as they can comfortably go on each side. Repeat three times, slowly, then close your eyes to rest for one breath. Next, open your eyes and move them slowly in a clockwise circle three times, and then a counterclockwise circle three times, closing your eyes to rest for one breath between directions.

NIGHTTIME HIP OPENER

Start by sitting on your bed with your legs stretched out. Then bend your knees, bringing the soles of your feet together, and spread your knees out to the sides. Hold on to your feet. (If you have tight hips, sit on your pillow.) Allow your knees to relax toward the bed, and breathe.

SLEEP SALUTATION

Lie on your back in *Savasana* (see page 129), palms facing up. Bring your awareness to your face. Scrunch it up tightly, and then release it. Then bring your awareness to your arms, lifting them up slightly off the bed, squeezing them tightly and clenching the hands, and then release them down. Then tense the muscles in the legs, and release them. Next, bring awareness to your head, imagining it softening and melting into the bed. Repeat this with each body part—shoulders, arms, chest, torso, abdomen, hips, legs, and feet—until you feel all of the tension has left your body.

RESOURCES

Books

CLASSICS

These classic books written by yoga luminaries are the foundations of a personal yoga library.

Autobiography of a Yogi, Paramahansa Yogananda

Be Here Now, Ram Dass

Bhagavad Gita: The Song of God, Swami Prabhavananda and Christopher Isherwood

Light on the Yoga Sutras of Patanjali, B.K.S. Iyengar

Light on Yoga, B.K.S. Iyengar

The Yoga Sutras of Patanjali: A New Edition, Translation, and Commentary, Edwin F. Bryant

YOGA PHILOSOPHY

These books are recommended for further reading on yoga philosophy.

The Deeper Dimension of Yoga, Georg Feuerstein

The Heart of Yoga, T.K.V. Desikachar

Krishnamacharya: His Life and Teachings, A.G. Mohan and Ganesh Mohan

Yoga and the Quest for the True Self, Stephen Cope

Yoga Mind, Body & Spirit, Donna Farhi

PHYSICAL YOGA PRACTICE

Learn more about a physical yoga practice in these recommended books.

40 Days to Personal Revolution, Baron Baptiste

Jivamukti Yoga: Practices for Liberating Body and Soul, Sharon Gannon and David Life

Kundalini Yoga, Shakta Kaur Khalsa

Power Yoga: The Total Strength and Flexibility Workout, Beryl Bender Birch

Relax and Renew: Restful Yoga for Stressful Times, Judith Hanson Lasater

Yoga Anatomy, Leslie Kaminoff

Yoga: The Poetry of the Body, Rodney Yee and Nina Zolotow

Yoga: The Spirit and Practice of Moving into Stillness, Erich Schiffmann

Yoga for Wellness: Healing with the Timeless Teachings of Viniyoga, Gary Kraftsow

Websites

These outlets for yoga overviews, news, and opinions offer many discoveries to the Web-surfing yogi.

ElephantJournal.com

With a focus on mindful living, this site offers yoga news, philosophy, and tips for incorporating yoga into everyday life.

HuffingtonPost.com

Visit the Healthy Living section for trends, news, and articles related to yoga practice.

YogaDork.com

Follow the latest in pop-culture yoga news with a humorous touch.

YogaJournal.com

This respected resource provides details on the practice, history, and philosophy of yoga.

Yoga Gear and Supplies

These companies carry or specialize in yoga-inspired clothing and gear. Each has online retail stores for easy accessibility.

Athleta

Gaiam

HuggerMugger

Lucy

Lululemon

Manduka

Prana

REI

Target

Zobha

Online Yoga Classes

These websites offer online classes for all skill levels and styles, for those who can't get to a class or would like some guidance with their home practice.

YogaGlo.com

Search for online yoga classes by teacher, style, level, or time.

YogaToday.com

Discover one-hour classes with a wide variety of styles and teachers.

MyYogaOnline.com

Browse by style, teacher, level, and length of class.

YogaVibes.com

Stream yoga classes and watch yoga videos.

INDEX